A SON'S JOURNEY

FROM PARKINSON'S DISEASE CAREGIVER TO ADVOCATE

IN MEMORY OF MY MOTHER SHARON
BY
DR. GEORGE M. ACKERMAN

Copyright ©2024 George M. Ackerman

All rights Reserved.
No part of this book may be reproduced in any form or by an electric or mechanical means, including information storage and retrieval systems, without permission in writing by the publisher, except by reviewers, who may quote brief passages in review.

ISBN: 979-8-9904489-1-9 (Paperback Edition)
ISBN: 979-8-218-40663-9 (Hardcover Edition)
ISBN: 979-8-9904489-3-3 (Ebook Edition)
ASIN: B0CX1HB8VJ (Kindle Edition)

TogetherForSharon®

https://www.togetherforsharon.com

Praise

A poignant tribute to a remarkable woman by an incredibly loving son. Like Dr. George Ackerman, I look forward to creating a future where future generations are spared the indignity of Parkinson's disease.
Ray Dorsey, MD, David M. Levy Professor of Neurology, University of Rochester, Author, Ending Parkinson's Disease

An honest from-the-heart true telling of what a family goes through in dealing with a neurodegenerative disease. We all have our own unique journey, but we are here for one another. This book is completely relatable as George went through this journey, as I did with my father who had Parkinson's.
Gary Keating, Author and Founder of Caring for Caregivers Support Group, fifteen years with Parkinson's.

A heart-wrenching story of the love of a devoted son for his mother, and how their life together was cut short due to Parkinson's disease. George Ackerman shares his journey as a care partner turned advocate who has taken his grief and channeled it into an instrument for raising awareness. This book is the story of one family's loss, but it is us who gain from his efforts and determination to end this disease forever.
Esther Labib-Kiyarash, MSHA, Person with Parkinson's and Ambassador for the Parkinson's Foundation

Reading this book allows you to understand the devastation of losing a parent to Parkinson's. Through George's example as a selfless, tenacious advocate for those who are still battling through this disease, we are able to see how his experience as a caregiver is invaluable to anyone in a similar situation as he approaches the situation with compassion and unadulterated love for his mother.

Melissa Livingston, Creator of #parkinsonslookslikeme, Patient, Pontificator and Parkinson's Advocate

George has written an important, heart-wrenching account of his journey as a caregiver and activist in the Parkinson's community. He honors his mother and the millions of people throughout the world fighting Parkinson's disease. As someone who was diagnosed with PD fourteen years ago, I found this book an emotional roller coaster that will help Parkinson's patients, caregivers, families, and friends battle this disease.

George Manahan, Parkinson's patient, activist, and supporter.

Nothing can prepare those taking care of their loved ones with Parkinson's disease (PD) for the journey they will face. However, this book is a raw and genuine account of the rugged road traveled by a devoted son. The courage to go from caregiver to PD advocate worldwide is inspiring. This book will help prepare caregivers for what PD can throw at them.

Kristine Meldrum, Author, Parkinson's: How To Reduce Symptoms Through Exercise

It is often through adversity and difficulty that the paths of our lives are changed, not unlike a river whose course is altered during a massive storm. And in this book, *In Memory of My Mother Sharon*, you'll read how the storms of adversity altered the life direction of Sharon's son George. You will read of how George went from a well-educated professional to a Parkinson's disease caregiver, and ultimately to a tireless and fearless Parkinson's disease advocate! In this book, Geor also does a great job of shedding light on the side of Parkinson's that is often overlooked, that of the caregiver.

Mark Milow, Public Speaker, Parkinson's Advocate, Parkinson's Foundation Advisory Board member, Cohost, Making It Meaningful: The Podcast; Cohost, Unscripted: The Parkinson's Podcast

I was moved to tears by the devotion Sharon' son George showed in the face of this horrific disease. The book is not only a testament to his character but also a "guidebook" for anyone who is living with a Parkinson's patient. I will be sharing George's courageous story with my friends and family, particularly my wife who has been watching me deal with PD since 2012. God bless you, George. We need more people like you in the world!

Dan O'Brien, Founder and Patient Advocate, DOB Parkinson's Charity, Living with Parkinson's since 2012

In this book, George takes the curtain down to reveal his journey from son to caregiver and from caregiver to advocate. His energy is palpable through the pages and the stories, which unmask challenge, hope, and future opportunity.

Michael S. Okun, M.D., *Adelaide Lackner Distinguished Professor of Neurology; Executive Director, Norman Fixel Institute for Neurological Diseases, University of Florida Health*

Thank you, George—for not only remembering your Mom in such a kind and loving tribute but for creating and engaging a global community to remember those we've loved and cared for who too struggled deeply with the challenges of Parkinson's. You have lovingly built an extended family worldwide—a heartfelt tribe that brings advocacy to a new and heightened level and makes awareness for Parkinson's a top priority.

Deb Pollack, Founder, *Drive Toward a Cure for Parkinson's Disease*

George has eloquently articulated what it means to not only love someone with Parkinson's but also what it is to tirelessly care for someone with this insidious disease. Through George's honest accounts, readers will develop a relationship with George, and his beloved mother, as he takes them on a journey hallmarked with love, compassion, and bravery.
Margaret Preston, President, Power Over Parkinson's

This book is a heartfelt tribute from a wonderful son to his mother, as well as a source of comfort for anyone whose life has been touched by Parkinson's disease. George does a beautiful job sharing the journey many take on this disease path. Readers will be able to relate to George's journey and not feel alone.
Tom Seaman, Health Coach, Author, Speaker, Patient Advocate

I highly recommend this heart-touching book about Dr. George Ackerman 's caregiving experiences and the love between a mother and son. Dr. Ackerman has a fierce passion for Parkinson's disease awareness advocacy, to help find a cure and to help others!
Betsy Wurzel, Host of Chatting with Betsy, Passionate World Talk Radio

Dedication

In memory of Sharon Riff Ackerman
My Mother,
But more importantly, my best friend.

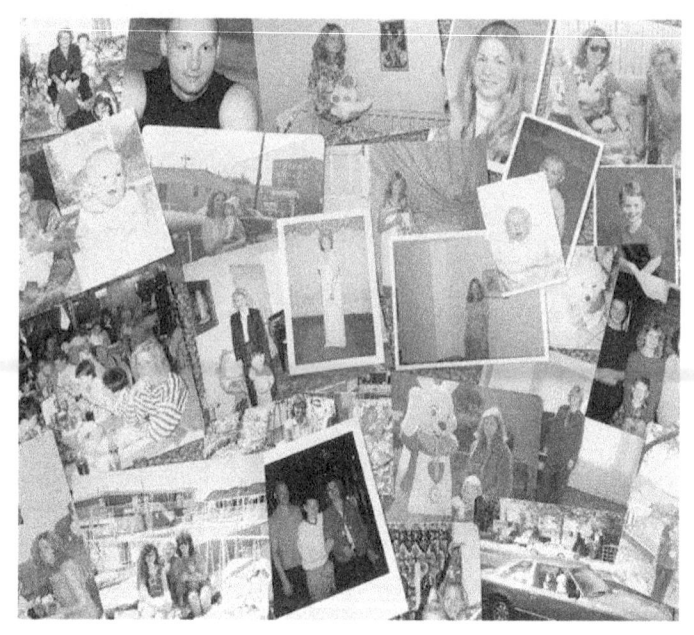

Table of Contents

Praise iii
Dedication vii
Introduction 1
Chapter 1 First Signs 6
Chapter 2 Symptoms, Associated Illnesses, and Treatments 15
Chapter 3 My Primary Caregiving 24
Chapter 4 Steadfast family Support: Partner 40
Chapter 5 Steadfast family Support: Children 55
Chapter 6 Trying to Find Good Aides and Caretakers 69
Chapter 7 Finally, Great Caregiving 79
Chapter 8 The Final Week 92
Chapter 9 Family and Friends Remember Sharon .. 101
Chapter 10 The Aftermath 110
Chapter 11 The Mission Forward 120
Chapter 12 Grateful To So Many 133
Appendices 144
About the Author 150

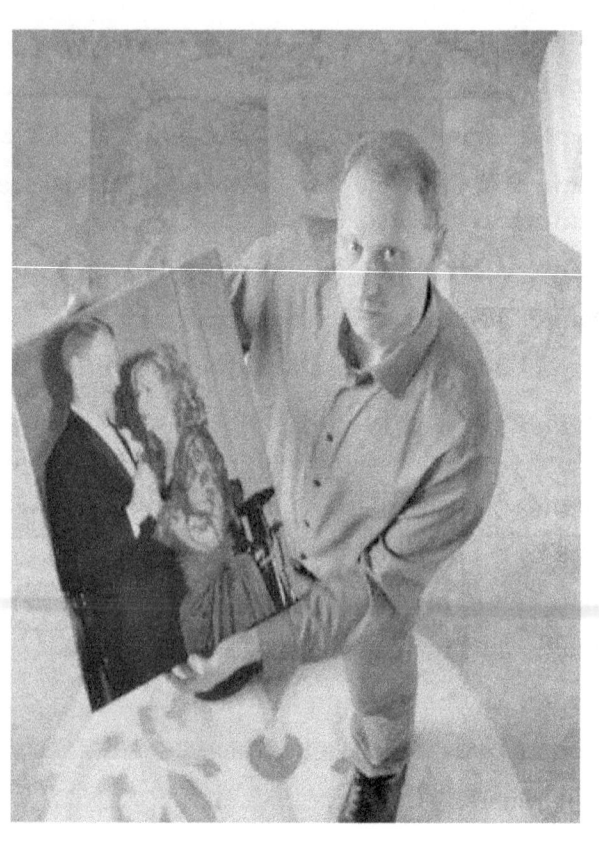

Introduction

This book is, first, a memoir of and praise for my mother, Sharon Riff Ackerman, who was my best friend through both our lives until her untimely death. The book is a heartfelt and often heart-wrenching recollection of the beginnings of her Parkinson's disease symptoms to the inevitable end. This book, too, is primarily for relatives and caregivers of those with Parkinson's.

However, I also want to reach those who are not aware of Parkinson's throughout the world. Until we ensure that others outside the local or regional Parkinson's community are made aware, a cure will be further from our grasp. Others, too, may find the book helpful, especially for those suffering from associated diseases.

My experiences with my mother and family are undoubtedly different from yours, but we all have similar feelings, questions, and thoughts. So, I share mine in this book. I hope my journey offers insights into yours. It is acceptable to recognize, admit, and face our painful, difficult, and sometimes contradictory feelings—and they are all completely natural. Through my recollections and journal entries, I want to help you with your own, asking and getting answers to questions and doing everything you can to help the sufferer and yourself.

The Purposes of This Book

So, painful as it has been, I've written this book with several purposes.

The first is to honor my mother, Sharon Riff Ackerman, who died too young at sixty-nine from Parkinson's disease (PD).

The second is to recount my experiences as her son dealing with her disease. This saga is admittedly for my release, maybe to continue to feel close to her, and possibly to exorcise my nagging feeling that, like many relatives and friends of PD sufferers, I could have done more. However, rationally, I know that wasn't possible.

The third purpose is to help sufferers, those diagnosed and living with Parkinson's, caregivers, family members, and friends to confront the disease.

The fourth is to comfort and assure them that their sometimes conflicting, often puzzling, and very often frustrated feelings are normal.

The fifth is to provide a guide and offer practical suggestions and resources for dealing with PD.

The sixth is to raise awareness of PD and vigorously support the search for a cure.

I've written to explain and teach, and I hope that other people and members of organizations will read my words as a plea and do something more. Over the years, I have sought every single opportunity: I consulted over twenty-five doctors with my mother to seek remedies for the disease and countless nurses and aides. I researched the entire medical field for a cure for Parkinson's. The responses, over and over, were always the same: "We don't know." "We can't do more." "We can't help any further." Most of the time, despite trying every expert, venue, area, topic, and resource and leading to hope, all my efforts led to nothing. And I felt like a failure. This book is a further cry for help.

My narratives and journal entries are heartfelt and tragic. They show, I hope, my great love and devotion to my mother. They express my feelings as I witnessed her decline because of

Parkinson's. Despite all my family and I did, I couldn't escape the recurring feelings of hopelessness and never having done enough. Admittedly, much of this book is hard to read, especially my account of the last year. But it was harder to live through—and that is why we need a cure.

Here are the steps and resources involved in my searches:

Research into the latest medical knowledge.

Opinions (often differing) of experts.

The best practical help at every stage.

Today, though, coming out of our darkness, a light of hope shines for so many others fighting Parkinson's. Medical breakthroughs are taking place, and hope for a cure becomes more real. Increasing awareness too is taking place. I continue to push the boundaries daily to reach those inside and outside the Parkinson's community worldwide. My message is unwavering and constant: we need to end PD now.

The Structure

This book is not meant as a medical tome—I do not have the credentials or knowledge—but an experiential one. The chapters are generally chronological, from the first signs to the gradual worsening and the final six months. It is an intimate, unflinching chronicle of the journey, primarily from my perspective. Yes, much is depressing, but also optimistic. I strengthened and kept discovering ever-greater resilience resources within myself to do what was necessary, although at steep costs to my physical and mental health.

Suggestions from my experience dealing with PD are included at the end of several chapters. The Appendices also contain more resources and information related to each chapter.

Many of the twelve chapters contain my journal entries that document my mother's decline, the steps I took to help her, and my feelings. To any PD relative or caregiver, I highly recommend journaling. It is not only cathartic but often, as if by magic, leads to ideas for contacts, further research, and solutions.

Progression

The journey was a very long one. I learned of Parkinson's in 2005, when, at my mother's first signs, my father, a physician, described the symptoms of possible Parkinson's. At the time, she started feeling abnormal and noticed areas of her body were rigid, unlike she had ever experienced, such as stiffness in her left arm. I thought the symptoms weren't bad for about thirteen years, but they accelerated in 2017. Today, I often wonder whether my mother either tried to hide her diagnosis so as not to burden me and the family or whether she was simply unaware. Or was the medical community not forthright and somewhat unsure as to the truth, speed of debilitation, and the ravages of this horrible disease? I wish my mother would have confronted it more directly from the first day.

My mother actively had Parkinson's for fifteen years. The last four were increasingly unpleasant, and the years became more intolerable as things worsened. The final seven months, June 2019 to January 1, 2020, were horrible for her and the entire family. And the last eight days of her life, from December 24, 2019, to January 1, 2020, were unspeakable.

I became the primary caregiver in 2019 and then hired a succession of aides, all of whom were disappointing. I saw I needed to take over as my mother's situation became more critical. It was during this time that I learned about the terrible toll of Parkinson's to caregivers on the mind, body, and soul.

Overall Purpose

This book is not meant as a wallow in misery or a chronicle of my sacrifices. I don't need or want these, nor do I want to subject readers to them. Neither is the purpose to gain praise for being a model son (if there is such a thing). I don't need this either. The many harrowing details and feelings I describe are meant to alert readers to the horrors of Parkinson's and to underscore its cruelty. I want to inform readers about the signs, prepare them, and emphasize the need for further, consistent research and advocating for a cure.

If the book is depressing, I understand. If it is informative, I'm glad. If it spurs you to act and contribute in any way(s) you are led to, I'm thrilled. We are all in this together.

www.togetherforsharon.com

Chapter 1: First Signs

When my wife Grether and I were dating, I used to joke that I had to excuse myself and call my mother. "Why?" Grether would ask. "To tell her how great you are!"

She would laugh and hug me. And that's how I felt about everything. When something was good, I wanted to tell my mother; when something was bad, I wanted to tell her. She was my best friend and confidante. I always listened to her wise counsel, and she never steered me wrong.

I'd shared with my mother the tribulations of dating and trying to find the right woman, a life partner who would understand me and with whom I could share everything. Just when I stopped looking and thought I would never find the right person, Grether came into my life.

My family moved to Florida in 1995. If we hadn't, I would never have met Grether. We met in the fall of 2010 when Grether was studying criminal justice, and I was working nearby. We discovered a mutual passion for helping others and a similar calling to the criminal justice field, which we were both studying. She worked with children, and I worked with victims of crime, both closely related to criminal justice.

With this shared love, we became good friends. But anything more was a slow start because I was busy working multiple jobs, and Grether was working, too. At one point, she saw my CV (which was over 100 pages) and casually commented when she read about my law degree, police officer training, and current PhD program that she liked redheads, lawyers, police officers, and scholars.

How could I refuse? And I thought, "Mom would love her."

We started dating. Not only did we have so much in common, but she was also extremely intelligent, easygoing, and beautiful. More importantly, Grether was and is a caring, kind, and beautiful person. (She certainly didn't know how much she'd have to support me during my mother's illness.) We had many long talks and very long phone calls late at night. I couldn't hide my joy, and after we started dating, I told my mother all about Grether. Her only slightly negative comment was about Grether's name: "An odd name . . . was it made up?"

I told her what Grether had explained to me. Although of Cuban descent, in which, as in many other cultures, babies are named after past relatives, her grandmother had created the name and told her it was "specially for you." And she was—and is special—a rare girl with a rare name—and the girl of my dreams.

My mother was very happy to see me so happy and excited to meet Grether. I knew that the woman I was captivated by had to be right; my mother would have to like her, and they would have to get along. Otherwise, it wouldn't work. But I was sure it would.

Three months after we started dating, in March 2010, I introduced them. I chose a small, older Chinese restaurant, my mother's favorite, close to her home. The walls were full of old-fashioned Chinese artwork, and the food was always fresh and delectable. It was a family-owned business, and the owners addressed my mother by her first name and hugged her. She introduced them to Grether and me. Smiling, they bowed slightly. And gave us the best corner table.

My mother looked elegant but casual: in a purple gem-encrusted shirt draped softly over her frame, matching eardrops, and black capri pants. I don't remember what Grether was wearing (I was too nervous). As they sat across from each other, both smiled, curious but shy. My mother remarked how much I had spoken about Grether since we met. "He talks of nothing else!"

Grether blushed.

My mother was relaxed, calm, and sweet and asked how we met, more about Grether's life and interests, and what she liked most about me. Grether was very forthcoming and, in turn, asked about my mother's life. They shared experiences like old friends, even though, at that early point, none of us knew where the relationship would go.

I sat back in awe and was jubilant. A good relationship with my mother for my potential partner—and I did believe Grether was *the* one—was critical in my life. They seemed like a perfect fit, and after only a few moments, it felt like they had known each other for years. Quickly, my mother came to love her as a daughter-in-law. Little did I know that Grether would prove to be the committed, wonderful, strong helpmate I needed during the terrible years of my mother's PD.

So, the next year, in 2011, Grether and I married in a wonderful and spectacular wedding. My mother looked radiant in a beautiful blue dress, bought especially for the occasion. From that point on, she and Grether couldn't stop smiling and hugging one another.

We moved nearby and saw my mother often for dinners, movies, shows, and even a concert by my mother's absolute favorite, Barry Manilow. I fondly recall us sitting in the National Car Rental arena in Sunrise, Florida, dancing from our seats to his "Copacabana."

Now I recall that as a child, when we lived in Brooklyn, I was forced to listen to his music as we drove throughout the city. But eventually, I got to enjoy the music, and now, whenever I put on a vinyl record of Manilow's, I'm back in those joyous times with my mother.

Grether and I saw my mother every Sunday and spoke several times daily.

In 2012, our daughter Brooke was born, in 2014 our son Joshua, and in 2017 our son Eli. My mother gloried in the grandchildren and loved giving them small gifts.

She was very happy that our first child was a girl because, as a mother of two boys, she always dreamed of a daughter and buying her dolls. The first gift she bought Brooke as a baby was a tickle-me Elmo doll (when you squeeze it, it giggles). Brooke was a serious baby, but when she saw my mother and the Elmo doll, she would smile brighter than any smile I ever saw.

With the boys, my mother always encouraged them to dance, sing, and enjoy life. She bought them coloring books and sat with them weekly while they colored. And she loved buying bubble kits and blowing bubbles with them, which always made them laugh as they tried to outdo each other with bigger bubbles. She always wanted them to be happy and gave them her complete love and total support. Some days, even now, I can see her blowing bubbles with the children in our backyard. I thought she would do this for years, but it was not to be because of Parkinson's.

My mother was very independent and strong-willed. She did not confide in Grether or me about her medical issues, although she told her friends. My father reached out when he heard from her friends that she did not feel well, but she never said exactly what it was. We had never heard of Parkinson's disease.

Maybe her independence was a result of her upbringing. Sharon had loving and supportive parents and remained close to her sister all her life. Her father, my grandfather George (whom I was named after), served honorably in the Army and was in D-Day. After the war, he worked for a jewelry company, then a dental concern, and later as a sanitation truck driver. In the Army, he discovered he had a heart condition, and during his rounds in the truck, he had a fatal heart attack.

Of course, this was a blow to his wife, my grandmother Pauline. But she rallied, working full-time at a department store, then at various office jobs, and raised her children at the same time. Pauline helped raise me as a child, too, and I remember her caring and fun—and discipline—in the same was that she had raised my mother, Sharon.

Sharon's independent spirit saw her through many tough times—as a teenager losing her father when she was sixteen, going to college, and getting a master's degree when her family culture valued other things for women, like having a family. After graduate school, as a substitute teacher, she taught kindergarten and first-grade children and eventually married my father, whom she met during college.

My father wanted to become a doctor but could only seek his goals if my mother sacrificed her career in education. And she did. She also sacrificed a lot for others throughout her life. After marriage, she gave up teaching to raise a family—my brother and me. She devoted herself completely to her children, giving me a wonderful, loving, attentive childhood and always stressing the importance of education. That is probably why I am successful in education now. I have several advanced degrees and teach at the undergraduate, master's, and doctoral levels. She was by my side through every graduation, every day I thought I would not make it through a program, and every one of life's journeys and challenges.

I believe I am only the man I am today due to my mother's sacrifices, and I am forever grateful. In addition to being my mother, she was my coach and mentor.

My parents were married from 1972 to 1995, twenty-three years. In 1995, they divorced, a blow to the family, but my mother carried on and devoted herself to her children and later grandchildren. Shortly after the divorce, we moved to Florida to be near her mother and sister.

We were happy for many years. But the first troubling signs were in 1999 and progressively became worse. In 2005, when she was in her early fifties, her left arm became rigid. I was very busy with law school, the police academy, my doctoral studies, and building my own family. But we spoke every day.

Then, in 2016, the symptoms became more serious. During everyday activities, for example, eating, she said her left arm hurt, and I noticed she was having trouble cutting her food. She would express frustration, but none of us was aware that it was Parkinson's disease. (I found out later from a relative that she may have been diagnosed at the very first signs in 1984, but she never mentioned or discussed them with me.)

We thought it was arthritis and brushed it off, never dreaming it would be something serious. She was still able to function, although I did help her cut food in restaurants. As she ate or dressed, her arm became stiff and rigid. After that, she started losing the ability to use her arm and hand on the left side of her body.

I became very concerned and asked her about this. She dismissed it, saying it was probably muscle cramps.

Then, I noticed other things. Her left hand trembled, and her movements became slower. At first, I rationalized these things as natural parts of aging—so little was known about her condition or how serious it would become. But as time went on, the symptoms worsened, and my curiosity turned into deep apprehension. I witnessed her daily struggles, from the simple act of tying her shoelaces to the challenging task of holding a cup of tea without spilling it when her hand shook.

My father, as an orthopedic doctor, knew about her symptoms. He did not specialize in Parkinson's but had many patients with it. He had noticed the indications: her mask-like face and the "cogwheel" rigidity of her wrist: when she moved it up and down, clicks could be heard.

As to the causes of my mother's Parkinson's diagnosis, medically, there is not 100 percent certainty. I suspect, though, it could have been due to the aging of her home, especially mold issues, termites, and bugs that plague many homes. The remedy, pesticide sprays, we are discovering today, could have been potentially harmful, as well as bug repellents and environmental factors.

My mother had gone to several doctors, and their tests confirmed the diagnosis of Parkinson's. In 1998, my father flew down from New York to take her to an expert Parkinson's disease doctor, hoping to gain some answers and enable her to get some relief. She was first put on dopamine in 2000.

The Parkinson's doctor radically changed the dosage of her medications, and this change caused dramatic side effects. It was likely the turning point that started her immediate decline.

She knew, too, that we had school, work, and a family, so she tried to handle her life and decisions in her own way. She didn't want to interfere in any of our lives and never wanted to be a burden to anyone. So, when she noticed the first signs, she did not come to us. Despite the signs, my mother did not look sick and was able to live a normal and independent life until the final three years, 2017 to 2020, when she came to depend totally on me and needed increasing support.

She faced her condition only when she had no other choice. This was after she had been diagnosed with Parkinson's and put on the medications.

One night in October 2017, I suddenly woke up at around 3:00 a.m. It was my father from New York. He was frantic and yelled that I needed to get over to my mother's house immediately. She had managed to call him in New York to beg for help. I rushed to her home and found her having a panic attack. That night changed our lives forever.

A neighbor of hers had called my father to let him know that, in the pitch black of night, my mother was outside, moving her furniture into the middle of the street.

As a police officer, I was trained for emergency calls but had never experienced one from my own family. I ran to my closet, threw on some clothes, and dashed out the door, worried and uncertain about what was going on, why, and what I would find when I arrived at my mother's house.

She lived approximately fifteen minutes from my home. There was no traffic, and as I approached her cul-de-sac, I noticed a shadowy female frantically moving furniture out of her home and screaming. I was not able to make out what she was saying. When I parked in the driveway, despite what my father had said, I was shocked to find that it was my mother and that she was not her normal self.

She seemed confused, agitated, and worried. I was also very scared for her and had no clue as to what I was dealing with, why, or how or who to contact to help her. I put my arms around her and tried to calm her down and assure her that everything would be okay. The only thing she said was that she was worried someone was going to harm her, and she was moving her items out of her house. I thought her belief may have been due to a sudden change in the Parkinson's medication. I finally succeeded in calming her down. I put her in a chair and gave her some tea. Then I moved everything back into the house.

Because of the severity of her behavior, I decided to take her to the hospital. I checked her in and put her in the hands of the medical staff. Then I left to go back to her home to pick up clothes in case she had to stay for some time. There, I was shocked again to find what is now one of the saddest memories I have ever had. As I entered Mom's bedroom, I noticed yellow post-it notes covering the bed and chairs. I looked closer and saw that each note had names of different relatives, friends, and pets of my mother throughout her life. Under each name was specified who was not alive, who did not live in Florida, and who may not have been nearby with her at the time.

Seeing all this made me cry, and I felt helpless. That day crushed my heart and soul. But I packed up some of my mother's clothes and went back to the hospital to be with her and find out what had happened. With everything that had transpired and what I'd seen in her room, I was very worried about the future and what was going to happen from there. No one, including me, of course, could have prepared for anything like this. It was an unknown territory, and I was in shock, worried, and very fearful about the uncertain future for Mom and our family.

In the hospital, my mother had an array of tests, and the diagnosis was a urinary tract infection. She was placed on medication and transferred to a rehabilitation center for a week. She hated being there, but the infection cleared up. After that night, though, I recognized that Parkinson's disease and dementia had set in and escalated, causing her delusions and hallucinations. Those post-it notes showed she didn't remember much about the family, and her furniture-moving attested to a succession of delusions.

It became apparent that she could no longer live by herself, and she needed care 24/7. This was the first time I ever really thought about or talked about the word "caregiver" because no one in my family had ever needed such help. But I had to face it. And, because of my great love for her, I knew I was up to the challenge.

The stay at the rehab facility also made our family aware that she strongly objected to living in a place like that or a home again. She begged me to stay with her in her home. This is where my journey began in a search for caretakers. We could not keep running over to her house to care for her, especially with the more difficult tasks like bathing. The hospitalization, the rehab, and her mental crisis marked a new chapter of her Parkinson's journey. The once vibrant woman I knew was slowly slipping away, a victim of the cruel grasp of Parkinson's.

As Grether and I and our family looked after Mom, we were thrown into the world of home care aides and long-term care. We started on an in-depth journey to learn what Parkison's was. From that night, everyday things continued to worsen and became especially severe over the final year before she passed on New Year's Day of January 2020.

Chapter 2: Symptoms, Associated Illnesses, and Treatments

The Tulip

For many years, tulips have had a special meaning for me. One evening, as Grether and I waited at the bar of our favorite restaurant for our table, I noticed a man sitting nearby with an intriguing lapel pin. It was a tulip—a red flower with four graceful points and two artistic green leaves twice as large, forming what I thought was a circle. I leaned over and commented on how aesthetic it was, especially the leaves.

He smiled. "Many people don't get it at first. The two leaves, with a line between them, are the initials P and D—they stand for Parkinson's disease. And the pin is a symbol of awareness and solidarity." I looked closer and indeed saw the letters PD.

"How did this come about?" I asked and introduced myself. He said, "I'm Greg," and held out his hand. "Well, I'll tell you. In 2005, the tulip was adopted as the official symbol of Parkinson's at the 9th World Parkinson's Disease Day Conference in Luxembourg, Belgium. However, it had been informally associated with the disease for more than 20 years before that.

"Wow," I said, and Grether pulled her chair closer.

Greg continued, "In 1980, a Dutch horticulturalist named J.W.S. Van der Wereld had Parkinson's. He developed a new red and white variant of the tulip and named it after Dr. James Parkinson, who first described the symptoms of the disease in 1817 in his *Essay on the Shaking Palsy*. So, the Dr James Parkinson tulip was adopted in 2005, as I said, and it is now universally known as the symbol for Parkinson's."

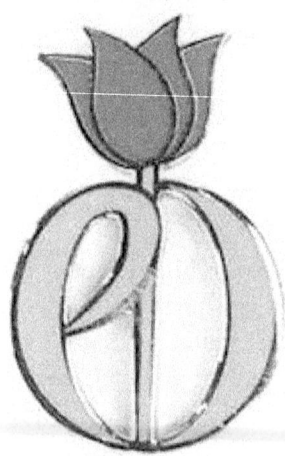

"What does it do?" Grether asked.

"It identifies everyone who may be suffering or have family and friends who have Parkinson's and binds them together, like members of a club wearing the same t-shirt. And more, it helps raise awareness about the disease and the need for additional and extensive research and shows support for everyone living with Parkinson's and their families globally."

"That's wonderful!" I said, and Grether dabbed at her eyes.

"And you?" I asked, "Not that I want to invade your privacy."

"Not me," Greg said, "but my mother."

Little did I know then that I would feel a special kinship with Greg. Six years later, I witnessed the first signs of Parkinson's with my mother.

The symptoms are frightening and sometimes subtle; many are common to other diseases. The primary symptoms are listed in other books (see Appendices), and I reiterate them here to highlight the major ones, especially those my mother suffered. Because of their subtleties and similarities to those of other illnesses, we weren't sure and determined we needed specialists' opinions.

Symptoms

The symptoms of Parkinson's disease can vary from person to person, and I and my family witnessed a number of these with my mother. They crept up from 2005 and became full-blown in 2016. Not everyone with Parkinson's disease will experience all these symptoms, and the progression and severity of symptoms can vary. Parkinson's is further complicated in treatment because the signs may vary and, at times, are entirely different in everyone diagnosed. For example, my mother had few external tremors but did have internal ailments.

The following list is not exhaustive, but the symptoms are common, and I witnessed them with my mother. I list them here so you may be alert to them.

Tremor: Typically, a resting tremor, is a rhythmic shaking or quivering of a
body part, often starting in the hands.

Bradykinesia (Greek "Brady" = slow, "kinesia" = movement) is a slowness of movement that is a hallmark of PD. Everyday tasks, like walking, getting up from a chair, or writing, become more difficult.

Muscle rigidity: The stiffness or inflexibility of the muscles can cause pain and limit the range of motion.

Postural instability: Impaired balance and coordination lead to difficulty maintaining an upright posture and an increased risk of falls.

Changes in speech: Soft, slurred, or monotonous speech and speech patterns.

Writing changes: Handwriting may become smaller and more cramped, known as micrographia.

Loss of automatic movements: Difficulty with unconscious movements, such as blinking, smiling, or swinging arms while walking.

Non-motor symptoms: Parkinson's disease can also involve non-motor symptoms like depression, anxiety, sleep disturbances, constipation, and cognitive changes.

Irritability, anger, violence: Behavior changes such as these may occur in the later stages and often result from the frustrations of the illness and loss of functions.

Although my mother had many of these symptoms for many years, even as far back as 1999, it wasn't until 2016 that I noticed more specific things—her trouble using her left arm, slower movements, trouble tying her shoelaces, inability to hold a cup of tea without spilling it. She didn't show every sign of the disease, as listed here. But it seemed like every time we identified and tried to focus on one issue, another would show up. Some of her problems were so debilitating that most days, she cried all day.

The Five Stages of PD

Today, medical authorities agree on five stages of PD. The duration can be short or long. Mother suffered through them all, from 1999 forward. Despite whatever we did and wherever we took her for consultation and treatment, my family and I watched helplessly. As you would expect, the stages became progressively worse.

In the first stage, the symptoms are mild and hardly interfere with everyday living. If anything, symptoms may show on one side of the body, such as tremors. Sometimes, the person experiences detrimental changes in posture, walking, and facial expressions.

In the second stage, the symptoms become a little worse. Both sides of the body may become rigid, or the person may experience aggravated tremors. Sometimes, the neck and torso are affected. There's more trouble walking, too. The person can still live alone but has difficulty with daily activities.

In the third stage, the person is more prone to losing balance and falls. The person can still perform daily tasks, but they are even more difficult. This stage is considered "mid-stage" by experts, who label the disability mild to moderate, even though the person can still function independently.

The symptoms worsen in the fourth stage. Walking and standing can still take place, but canes or walkers are often used for steadiness and alleviation of falls. Living alone is impossible now; people need help with daily activities and tasks.

In the fifth stage, the most debilitating, leg stiffness may prohibit standing or walking. The person lives in a wheelchair or bed and needs round-the-clock care.

Associated Illnesses

Again, this discussion is not exhaustive but relates to my experiences with my mother. For more thorough descriptions, see Appendices and the Internet.

Dementia

Parkinson's can bring on other problems, such as dementia. My mother had late onset dementia. Possible symptoms of dementia:

Difficulty completing familiar tasks, for example, making a drink or cooking a meal.

Problems communicating: difficulty with language, forgetting simple words, or using the wrong ones.

Disorientation: for example, getting lost or disoriented on a previously familiar street.

Mood changes: sudden and unexplained changes in outlook or disposition.

Memory loss: repeated questions, even after answers are supplied.

Personality changes: a previously calm and unruffled person becoming irritable, suspicious, or fearful.

Loss of initiative: progressively less interest in starting something or going somewhere.

As patients age, late-stage dementia symptoms tend to worsen.

In addition to Parkinson's, my mother suffered from dementia towards her final year. I noticed many signs. I do remember delusions and hallucinations four years earlier when she went to a university study. I'm sorry to say that this study was a monumental failure. The doctor drastically changed her medicines, and that was the beginning of her immediate health decline.

She was agitated much of the time, fearful, and scared that individuals were harming her or would do so. She "saw" family members who lived in other states and family who had passed and asked repeatedly for her mother, who had passed decades before.

One instance haunts me still today. When my daughter Brooke was nine, she and I were in my mother's room. Mom was resting with her eyes closed, and we were keeping her company. She looked like she had dozed off, but she suddenly awoke and was enthusiastically repeating Brooke's name and hugging a towel. Mother kept repeating my daughter's name, saying how much she loved her.

Even though Brooke was in the room, my mother believed the towel was my daughter. Brooke didn't understand what was happening, but I cringed, fearing the worst, and, wanting to help, held my mother's hand. I explained that Brooke was right there, but my mother didn't understand. I felt completely frustrated and wanted to find someone, somewhere, to help us all, but I could not.

After the university debacle, we took my mother to a psychologist and then a psychiatrist for her dementia. Neither helped, nor did the medications she was given.

I videotaped and photographed many episodes of her because, first, I could hardly believe them myself, and second, I hoped that if I showed the videos to doctors, they might magically have a remedy. They did not.

It pained me terribly to see her like this. But I could only hold on, keep seeking help, elusive as it was, and answer her incessantly repeated questions, reassuring her of her fears and soothing her in her hallucinations.

Before my mother showed signs of dementia, I never even knew it existed. I wish I could have answers or advice for others who suffer from this malady.

Dyskinesia and Dystonia

As the PD progressed, my mother also developed other diseases, among them dyskinesia and dystonia. Dyskinesia is characterized by low magnesium levels, muscle fatigue, less control over voluntary movements. and especially involuntary muscle movements, like tics and twitches. Dyskinesia can go from a slight tremor of the hands to an uncontrollable upper-body movement or lower-body trembling.

Mother showed signs of dyskinesia, with involuntary muscle contractions that caused repetitive twisting movements of her body. These movements took place randomly and were unrelated to any other cause, such as hunger or lack of sleep. Due to dyskinesia, she swayed her body, moved her head, and fidgeted significantly.

Dyskinesia is mainly caused by medications, such as the long-term use of Levodopa in Parkinson's disease and the use of antipsychotic drugs. Mom was taking Levodopa, and doctors told me that this medication can cause dyskinesia.

Dyskinesia caused by brain injury, such as a vascular event (stroke) or other brain damage, is less common. Movement symptoms typically start as minor shakes, tics, or tremors. The symptoms also include abnormal facial, mouth, and tongue movements, including involuntary lip-smacking, repetitive lips pouting, and tongue protrusions.

Dystonia manifests as involuntary muscle contractions, slow, repetitive movements, or abnormal postures. It often involves muscle stiffening, twisting, and abnormal sustained positions, such as an arm in an awkward position or head tilting sideways. When Mom showed these symptoms, she always seemed uncomfortable, as I could see from her facial grimaces, and they often interrupted her daily activities.

I researched furiously and discovered some recommendations:

Ease of stress. Stress can make dyskinesia worse. Relaxation methods include massage, yoga, meditation, reading, or talking to a friend.

Physical activity—exercise, walking, bike riding, even boxing. These have many benefits for combating Parkinson's.

Speech therapy, physical therapy.

Change in medication dosage.

Change in diet to more healthy foods that can minimize the side effects of medication.

Continuous drug infusion.

Deep brain stimulation.

Fibromyalgia

Fibromyalgia is a disorder characterized by widespread musculoskeletal pain, accompanied by fatigue, sleep, memory, and mood issues. Researchers believe that fibromyalgia amplifies painful sensations by affecting the way the brain processes pain signals. This condition can be hard to understand, even for healthcare providers. Its symptoms mimic those of other conditions, and there aren't any actual tests to confirm the diagnosis. As a result, fibromyalgia is often misdiagnosed and remains challenging to treat.

Symptoms:

Pain in the muscles and bones (musculoskeletal pain)

Areas of tenderness in many areas of the body

Pain or a dull ache in the lower belly

General fatigue

Trouble sleeping

Sleeping for long periods without feeling rested (nonrestorative sleep)

Headaches

Dry eyes

Cognitive disturbances, such as trouble focusing or paying attention

Depression, from mild to severe

Anxiety, from mild to severe

Bladder problems, such as interstitial cystitis.

Mom suffered terribly from fibromyalgia. Back pain was her main complaint, but she also described it as pain throughout her entire body. And she often cried.

In addition to Parkinson's and dementia, we struggled to help her with her pain issues. She tried medications, psychology, pain management, and even medical marijuana. None of it worked. As with my mother's other maladies, before she told me about fibromyalgia, I never even knew it existed.

Sharon had Parkinson's disease, dementia, dyskinesia, dystonia, and fibromyalgia. It was tough to concentrate on or isolate just one of these illnesses to find help for her because so many issues surfaced almost simultaneously. It was so saddening, frustrating, and depressing. But Grether and I explored every symptom, and I researched them thoroughly, trying to gain as much information as possible as quickly as I could. I was looking for alleviation and—dare I hope—a cure.

These associated illnesses are well-recognized in the PD community. An image, "The Parkinson's Iceberg," graphically depicts the constellation of illnesses and what most others don't see. As Sharon's disease progressed, more of these symptoms and illnesses became evident.

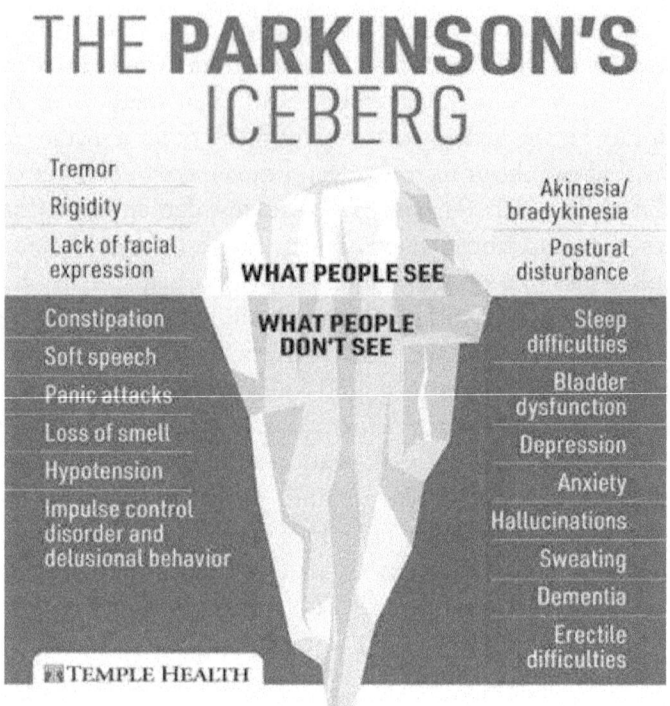

Illustration credit: Temple Health.

Treatments

Treatments vary with the individual and condition. I recommend that anyone seeking treatment consult their medical professional(s).

What follows is our experience—Grether's and mine. Despite her busyness with the children, the house, and her studies, she accompanied me to every doctor's appointment, investigated every new treatment, and continued steadfastly in her entire interest and support.

The major methods we pursued included the following:

1. Physicians: We reached out to numerous doctors but never seemed to get the answers we needed because there was no cure. They assessed Mom's individual needs and recommended strategies tailored to her condition, but none were truly effective enough as her condition became worse.

We visited over twenty doctors, and they all said she was doing well, that she would not die from Parkinson's disease, and that many studies showed others like her would not die.

But we had yet to receive helpful answers from doctors. The answers I repeatedly received were "We don't know," "We can't do more," and "We can't help any further." I had to conclude that doctors are no help because they cannot assist with Parkinson's disease at all.

2. Medications: Prescribed by physicians, Parkinson's disease is often managed with medications to control symptoms, such as tremors, rigidity, and slowness of movement. Different types of medication can be prescribed based on the specific needs of the individual. But, as recounted in Chapter 1, when my mother's medication was changed, the change affected her radically, and that led to her breakdown on the lawn and hospitalization.

Medicines never did help Mom's Parkinson's . . . or maybe the doctors could not determine what really would have helped her. As I've emphasized, they all said different things and prescribed medications in different amounts, but nothing ever seemed to help. It seemed like they were defining experimentally because they didn't know what would work. I learned more about medicines and taking care of my mother than I should have ever learned in a lifetime.

In the final year, we had a wonderful nurse who set up a pill box and schedule, which was helpful.

However, no one—neither doctors nor we—knew what medicine would help. Seeing so many pills, even though I had no medical training, somehow, I knew they could not be safe for anyone. Without them, though, she may not have survived at all, even though she did not endure for long. The vividness of my mother's condition was a major impetus for me to start the foundation TogetherForSharon® (http://www.togetherforsharon.com) for greater awareness and more research toward a cure.

For Parkinson's, she took Levodopa and Sinemet. For dementia, she took Namzaric and mirtazapine, which did not help. Also, she had terrible constipation and took Fiber, Dulcolax, and nurse-initiated enemas for that and significant pain, as well as a lot of Tylenol/Advil.

She took other medicines, too, all under the care of doctors, but again, none seemed to work. I saw bags and bags of medicines, one from this doctor and another from that. They had never coordinated into a team approach, so it is possible that the medicines worked against each other and even exacerbated her condition.

3. Physical therapy: For a person living with Parkinson's, working with a physical therapist can help improve mobility, balance, and overall strength. The therapist can provide exercises and techniques to manage specific Parkinson's symptoms. If you use one, ensure they are credentialed and familiar and experienced with the symptoms and the procedures.

Saturdays were my only day to relax for a couple of hours. One Saturday, I was dropping off groceries at my mother's when I thought I could take a day off from the chaos. The physical therapist confronted me at the door and said that Mom needed to be put into a mental facility immediately. The therapist could not get her to follow directions, and because of her associated illnesses, she couldn't move her body in the ways directed to do the needed exercises. And more: Her delusions and hallucinations caused her mental instability, which interfered with her ability to concentrate on exercises or even follow the directions.

At the physical therapist's report, I called my father, mother's doctor, and a healthcare coordinator and asked for advice. A long-term hospice was recommended. When I contacted the administrator, she seemed reassuringly understanding and supportive. So, we entered Mom.

But, for some baffling reason, with end-of-life diseases, physical therapy is not allowed. My mother still had hope and constantly repeated that she would not give up because she wanted to see my kids grow up and someday be at my daughter's wedding. However, the moment Mom was not allowed to have physical therapy, her body started shutting down. She became chronically sad and lost hope.

Movement was the only thing she had left, and they took it away. Yes, her body broke down, likely due to the disease and the numerous medicines she took. After she passed, I cleared out her home and discarded many large garbage bags of drugs. It still gnaws at me—was she even given the appropriate medications? Each doctor said something different. Did she take each medicine on the right day and time? Did the aides we hired provide the medication promptly and properly when I was absent?

There were so many medications, and they were prescribed in such high volumes and dosages. I believe the medications hurt my mother and quickened her decline. Ironically, as I've said, and it eats at me still, I was told by many medical professionals that one does not die of Parkinson's; one dies with it. But my mother was healthy, independent, and able to live normally until 1999. With all the medications and treatments, her health rapidly declined, and for that, none of us was prepared or could ever be.

4. **Occupational therapy:** Occupational therapists can assist in finding adaptive strategies and devices to maintain

independence in daily activities, such as dressing, eating, and writing. After the night I rushed Mom to the hospital, she had some occupational therapy for a few weeks at the rehab center. She was given writing instructions, but her hand shook, and she often couldn't hold a pen because of cramping. So, the therapy was ineffective.

5. **Speech therapy:** Speech and language therapists can help address speech and swallowing difficulties that may arise with Parkinson's disease. We engaged a speech therapist only in the final months. Mom had started to slur words and lose her speaking ability, so by that time it was too late.

6. **Supportive care**: With medical interventions, emotional support and assistance with daily tasks can be invaluable. Supportive care is provided by professional caregivers, support groups, or counselors to manage the emotional impact of the disease. We tried a psychologist at one point, but Mom did not like her and maintained she didn't understand. I also went with Mom a few times but felt my wife and family helped my mother more than a stranger did. As I kept learning, I understood that some healthcare professionals specialize in Parkinson's disease, and I explored more possibly appropriate methods for my mother's specific situation.

7. **Other therapies:** I wanted to try pet therapy, having read some promising reports for daily activities and anxiety. However, the specific program I was interested in had been terminated, so we never had that opportunity. It would have done Mom some good because she loved animals. Her first dog, when she was a teenager, was a dachshund named Baron, and when we lived in Brooklyn, she had a bichon frisé named Teddy. He looked like a stuffed animal, and I loved him. Much later, she used to pet sit for my dog, Jaxx, and two cats, Leo and Romeo, when I was in law school and unable to watch them for long stretches.

Pets helped Mom and me through many years. As anyone with pets knows, they are a great comfort and solace—and excellent listeners. I am a big believer in animal therapy, and even in Mom's last few months, she wanted me to get her another pet to keep her company. We never had that opportunity, though, because of her rapidly declining health from Parkinson's. She also could not care for a pet at that point, so it probably would have been another area I would have to cover. I could not commit to this added responsibility because all my time was dedicated to caring for her.

This recap reflects my experience and constant efforts to help my mother. Reading, researching, and speaking with people, I tried everything I could think of so that I would never regret not taking all opportunities to try something else. We took her to Parkinson's doctors and neurologists, massage therapists, psychiatrists, pain management specialists, and movement specialists, and we even got her medical marijuana. Looking back today, I would have done nothing differently. No other areas, even those I see today, would have been effective for our attempts—except for a cure.

8. **Medical Marijuana:** I give this topic a separate section because it is more controversial than other treatments, and I want to alert readers especially to it. In our experience, it was like the Wild Wild West.

I work in the law enforcement field, so even applying for a medical marijuana license was a questionable decision. But I was eager to do it because, in 1999, when her symptoms first started appearing, marijuana might have been my mother's last hope for some relief from her pain and suffering for decades from Parkinson's, dementia, and fibromyalgia.

In the United States, the **Controlled Substances Act** bans the use of cannabis. But in Florida, the Medical Marijuana Legalization Initiative, which went into effect in 2016, provides that patients with debilitating medical conditions can use medical marijuana for their symptoms. The first step is applying for a license, so we decided to do it as a last hope.

There are strict rules and procedures, so, we applied for a state license. It was not an easy task because, by some strange laws, doctors and dispensary people could not communicate with each other. No one could determine the dosage, and there was no time for a test trial. Applying for a license entailed fee upon fee upon fee, endless paperwork, and interminable waiting. But after three months, the license finally arrived. I feared it was almost too late.

We had to see the medical marijuana doctor first. He just seemed to guess as to the recommended dosage, and I hated subjecting my mother to an "experimental" recommendation. After the doctor gave me a prescription, we went to the dispensary.

The dispensary was cash-only and, at first, seemed very shady. However, the place looked strangely like a bank. It was spotless and beautiful, with wood partitions surrounding large wooden desks and all items placed in glass containers. It reminded me of a jewelry store because security guards were at the front door and the main waiting area. The armed guard at the entrance kept surveying everything, so we felt safe. In one corner stood a glass-enclosed case, where t-shirts were displayed, decorated with the store's name. Rather odd! I thought.

You wait outside until you are called, as if waiting to open a checking or savings account. We watched the people who were leaving, and they seemed happy. Grether and I squeezed hands; I won't deny that we were excited.

When our name was called, we entered a smaller room and stood in front of a counter like in a pharmacy. The man behind the counter nodded and stretched out his hand. I gave him the prescription, which was more like a guess from the doctor.

The dispensary clerk placed in my hand a little bottle of the pills and a small bottle of liquid that was specified on the doctor's sheet. However, no one could provide specific directions for the dosage. I worried that it would not work.

When we got home, with caution and holding our breaths, we first gave Mom half a pill. It did nothing. Then I gave Mom a full-strength pill. She slept all night, but the next day was groggy, and we suspected that even one pill was too much. We also tried liquid from the dropper bottles and could only guess at the dosages. With too much, she was so high she became agitated, upset, and sad and tipped over in her wheelchair. And marijuana is supposed to stimulate appetite, but it didn't for Mom. She continued to lose weight, even though I kept buying her favorite foods.

Maybe better communication between the doctor and dispensary—and us—could have helped. Medical marijuana may have helped others, but it did not help Mom, and her health was worse every day. Yet again, another hope faded.

Was it right or wrong to see so many doctors and specialists? I do not think so. We needed to exhaust any and every possible treatment that could possibly help her.

Chapter 3: My Primary Caregiving

Maybe it was foolhardy and egoistic, but I wanted to be my mother's primary caregiver. I worked as an attorney, police officer reservist, and professor of criminal justice and law. My family has always been my priority, followed by my education and work. However, when Mom's health declined rapidly, I was shocked. Despite my many activities, I reorganized my life to care for her and gave her my utmost attention. She would have done the same for me.

I kept a journal during the last year of my mother's Parkinson's battle. Aside from all the research and physical steps and actions I took, keeping the journal was how I dealt emotionally with it. It helped some . . . although it also constantly reminded me of the horror of it all. But my journal probably also kept me at least a little steady and sane to continue to do whatever I could for her. Here I will share journal entries in this chapter and the subsequent ones.

Some of the issues I talk about in this chapter were touched on earlier, such as Mom's delusions. But the context is different in each place—earlier, the delusions illustrate the horror of Parkinson's; here, they show how they affected my caregiving.

From the time I took over, I felt lost, confused, and frightened that I could not control her future. But I promised myself that I wouldn't give up and that, with Grether's help, I would exhaust every means available to assist and save Mother. But as I've said, I often felt as though I failed.

I found out quickly that caring for someone with Parkinson's disease takes a toll on the caregiver. As a caregiver, I mirrored many of my mother's issues—struggles with health, physical well-being, and mental fitness. I developed acid reflux, was exhausted much of the time, and felt at my wit's end.

As a son, it was my dream to be able to buy a brand-new home for my mother. I was finally able to do just that, but it came many years after we had moved to Florida and at a significant cost. From 1990, we'd had a two-story summer home in Boca Raton, Florida. In 1995, Mom took my brother Andrew and me from Brooklyn, New York, to the Florida home to join the family—her mother, Pauline, sister Ellen, and Ellen's son, my cousin Adam. I was also scheduled to begin college at a Florida university, starting my higher education and career. So, we moved to Boca Raton, Florida, and lived a block away from the relatives.

Mom lived in the Boca Raton house from 1995 to 2019; I left for law school in 2001, and Andrew moved away shortly afterward. The house was beautiful but had decades of issues—termites, mold, and many other problems because of deterioration, and I was sure it was unsafe. Mom lived alone by then, never had much help, and did everything independently. She didn't ask or tell me much about the house, and I never realized how bad it had gotten after so many years.

I completed college and eventually married. The Boca Raton house was 20 minutes away from where my family and I lived at the time, and Mom had begun having symptoms of Parkinson's. I wanted to be much closer to her because I knew I would need to be there for her more and more as the disease progressed.

So, I "rescued" her from the old house, and Mom finally agreed to let us buy her a brand-new home in Delray Beach, Florida, only a community away. It was a one-story, more accessible for her to get around in, and only five to eight minutes from where we lived (my wife and I, the kids, and my mother-in-law). I could rush over any time, day or night, if Mom needed anything, and it was a challenge and commitment I wanted to take on.

She was very excited. The home was sparkling new, and she chose everything to go in it, from the sinks to floors to furniture and decorations. She was like a kid in a candy store.

The house in Delray Beach took a year to build, and we moved her there in 2019. It was a dream home—four bedrooms, everything brand new. It had a large backyard on a manmade lake and inside a big-screen theater-like television, on which she loved to watch her favorite movies. We were all lifelong movie and television fans and enjoyed many hours in the "theater."

After she moved in, I imagined her enjoying the lake view and relaxing for years to come. I thought she would have ten years or more, but little did we realize the time would end too quickly. We were unprepared, and neither Grether nor I could have ever believed she would pass so fast. All her health issues, as I've said before, were side effects of the massive amounts of drugs she took for Parkinson's, and they affected her quickly—neurologically, mentally, and physically.

In 1996, Mom's health took a turn for the worse, and the disease rapidly escalated. This was after her trip to the Parkinson's trial for medicine, which we hoped would help but did not. As Parkinson's became more evident, even though she still lived in Delray, Mom, my wife, and I discussed moving her again, this time into a home we would build in Boca Raton. With three kids, my mother-in-law, two cats, and a dog, Mom would still have a place, and we had a room designed specifically for her.

We followed through, paid the deposit, and started to build. But Parkinson's claimed her in early 2020 before we even finished building the home. It was too late to cancel the contract.

However, Grether and I moved the family in once the house was finished. But I was also sick and heartbroken, recognizing that if we lived in this new larger home in Boca

Raton built for Mom and our family, the room meant only for her would be empty forever. Even today, it still haunts me as I write this sentence.

The Search Continues

As a caregiver, I had no experience but relied on my intuition—and, of course, the mountains of research and consultations with so-called experts, all to determine what was best for Mom. I couldn't handle many of her manifestations. Most nights, she was up 24/7, crying and voicing hope at the same time, but her health was constantly deteriorating. There were many other short-term and ongoing crises. I wanted to do more but wasn't equipped and suffered too as the caregiver.

We took her to over fifteen neurologists who (supposedly) specialized in Parkinson's disease, and they all came to the same conclusion I'd heard so often. They would deliver the words with godly authority: "You do not die from Parkinson's disease; you die with it." And they usually added that most PD patients live into their eighties or even nineties. To this day, we are not sure, and I am still shocked that she passed at the young age of sixty-nine.

However, I had heard of a new program in Florida, a long-term hospice-type group called Reliance (pseudonym). They would provide a nurse once a week to fill prescriptions, come to the house, give guidance, and be a phone call away when the nurse wasn't there. Unfortunately, hiring a private care company conflicted with the full-time aide (almost like a babysitter) I had hired for Mom through CaringComforters (pseudonym). If the caregiver did not follow the nurse's specific details, Mom would not have the correct medicines at the right time. I still don't know if her medications were administered correctly, and the possibility continues to frighten me to think about.

I needed help—I wasn't a medical doctor and did not have the expertise or even much knowledge about Parkinson's medications, dosages, or procedures for administering the medicines. But I felt somewhat better knowing a medical professional, the nurse, was now involved. And I felt a little more relief knowing that Mom was now living in the new home we built for her in the following community ten minutes away. I even set up a mini office in her house so I could be there and handle her affairs at any point. And the more I did for her, the closer I felt to her.

June 11, 2019

Mother calls from the new home and begs me to pick her up so she can live with me. She says that some man harmed her in the past when she was younger, and I explain that no one will hurt her now.

I have a headache and feel sick after her call. This is getting harder for her and me every day. I sit all day and night trying to think what I can do to help, but I still feel helpless even with everything I've done and am doing.

June 12, 2019

Mom calls at 7:00 a.m. and asks me again to take her away so she can live with me. She says that people are harming her, and I should watch the cameras I had installed day and night. I reassure her she is safe. Parkinson's does horrible things to the mind, and I see it firsthand now and feel helpless. I am sickened by not being able to do more.

I'm trying to live my life, but it's difficult, even if I escape for a few hours. I would be at work or with my children, eating dinner or trying to work out, when I'd get hysterical phone calls from my mother at all hours of the day. I'd drop everything to rush over to her place and never want to let her feel I was not a few moments away to rescue her. However, in reality, many times it was the disease that took over her mind, and I felt it took over mine as well.

June 22, 2019

Mother calls, frantic and screaming that a man is hurting a girl. I checked the video cameras in many places inside and outside her house, and no man has ever entered her home. Neither he nor the girl exists.

I ask her to calm down, but she says, "Please, move me to an apartment." She was living ten minutes away. I realized then that she probably thought she was back in New York, where she lived in an apartment as a little girl. Then she says she wants to live in an apartment in Century Village with 24/7 aides and a case manager. She's confused, her thoughts jumbled. I pursue the subject and ask why. She then says she's unsure and doesn't mention the man or girl.

June 30, 2019

I can do nothing but keep pursuing. Her mental health due to the disease declines rapidly and baffles me. I keep asking so many people to help and keep track of her doctors' appointments and take her to all of them.

I keep hearing those words from the physicians with such unimpeachable authority: "You do not die from Parkinson's; you die with it." We heard of many people with PD living even to the age of ninety. And, of course, we wanted to believe this pronouncement.

When I press, the authorities don't reply; they vanish or say I should ignore her and that it's the disease speaking. How can I "ignore" it? Her cries and pleas pull at me. I'm nagged by the feeling that more should be done, but especially without clearcut advice, I'm unsure what step might be next or what to do.

I am trying to avoid placing her in a care home, but even the best professional caregivers may not be able to assist with the mental challenges she faces daily. As this recent episode showed, Parkinson's, or possibly late-onset dementia, another new term I never heard of until now, is causing her delusions and hallucinations.

My mother would be horrified if she knew what she was doing to us. She's been the sweetest, friendliest, and most caring person I have ever met, and yet her personality is changing daily from this horrible disease. It's not only torturing me but my family as well. I cannot even express what it is like to go through, and I feel trapped in a box trying to figure something out. But I can do nothing at all. I'm learning more about a disease I wish I never heard about or had existed.

Mom's Delusions and Hallucinations

Mom's delusions and hallucinations were the toughest to handle. They caused Grether and me a great deal of distress. The illness made Mom feel constantly suspicious of people around her, and like she was attacked when she was not. It caused physical aggression, safety, social embarrassment, and stress, which forced more isolation.

Delusions

For example, she thought people were in the room, such as her parents (deceased) who were visiting her, but they weren't. She thought other family and pets were there, but they were dead. She felt that someone else was there and was an imposter pretending to be her friend and threatening to harm her, but no one was there or threatening her. She also thought items in the room—like pillows or chairs—were loved ones. And she talked to them and became furious when "they" didn't answer.

I recognized the delusions but didn't even want to tell her, fearing she would become more upset. And any explanation was not easy for her to understand. She was convinced of the truth of her delusions, and they were extremely painful for me to hear, see, and cope with.

She called 911 once, as I related, because she feared someone was breaking in. Another time, as I also recounted earlier, she moved her furniture out of her home onto the lawn because she thought people were coming to harm her. She sometimes thought her medicines were poisoning her and ignored them completely. This all caused me tremendous stress. No matter what I did or said, I couldn't find a way to calm her down or resolve the PD symptoms.

Hallucinations

Mom's intermittent hallucinations, too, caused me great concern. They also affected her with cognitive issues, depression, and sleep problems. She struggled with what was false and what was real. The episodes would generally take place when I was not with her. She would call me in a panic, cry out to me for help, and I would rush over. All I could do was hold and rock her. I had no answers. I also tried to show her how safe she was and pointed out the video cameras I'd installed so she knew I was always there, watching over her and protecting her.

Some of the scariest moments for me were when she thought her mother (my grandmother) was in the room. It was heartbreaking. I tried calming her down and telling her she was not crazy. Eventually, I had to remove her phone because she was calling 911 so often and reporting crimes that did not exist.

As Mom's dementia got worse, I became even more worried for her health and safety. She told me animals and deceased loved ones visited her daily. She told me of long talks with invisible people and recited her baby memories. Some days, the people she "visited" with were happier or sadder. She told me that her parents, who had passed decades earlier, were in a comfortable space. Other times, though, with terrifying hallucinations, she would cry and suffer attacks and was sure everyone was trying to harm her, especially the aides. She also called the police one night in fear. The new events were like nails, and every day, a hammer hit me repeatedly.

I was so troubled that I hardly knew what to do next to help her. But Grether and I agreed to try a psychiatrist for Mom. She wasn't too happy with this. She maintained vehemently that she wasn't insane and didn't want to go.

I tried to calm her down and explained we would speak to him. Finally, she agreed, and we met with the doctor. He asked about Mom's medical history and about what was happening. I explained the episodes, but Mom was frustrated and thought he didn't understand. He prescribed medicines, and we had the prescriptions filled, but Mom refused to take them, and we never went back.

As I've said, Mom took so many medications, and I never truly understood if they were contributing to the delusions and hallucinations and making them worse. As I've repeated, we went to many doctors, and even that psychiatrist, but we never felt we gained any answers to reduce her hallucinations or delusions. And they got worse. From the previously very positive and happy person she'd been, she became restless, fearful, angry, and continuously agitated.

These episodes led to tough talks about Mom going to a nursing home. My wife and I assumed the staff could provide more support than we could, but we didn't know if that was true. I worried that they might neglect her, so we finally agreed never to put her in a nursing home. I felt like I would be abandoning her if I left her at her house, but I also knew I was not equipped mentally or physically for all of this. I am glad we had the means to keep that promise to her. But it all took a heavy toll on me.

My Health

I sacrificed my health to ensure my mother had attention every moment. I didn't have the disease itself, but I felt like a secondary patient or, in a term I coined, a "secondary Parkinson's" who needed medical experts to guide me through the challenges. To me, secondary Parkinson's meant I did not have the Parkinson's physical symptoms, but I experienced all the signs my mother showed daily and the aftermath through her progression. The only problem was there was no support or help from another caregiver.

With power of attorney, I completely took over and assumed responsibility for all my mother's affairs in her final two years. I had to face callous decisions, and many were made without consulting her (I didn't want to make her even more upset), such as, much earlier, asking her not to drive any longer. With her driving, I feared she wouldn't remember how to brake and signal, much less remember where she was. I agonized over this decision many sleepless nights and knew not driving was further reducing her independence. But I had to decide in favor of her safety.

Mom had loved and enjoyed her independence most of her life. Taking away a person's car keys can leave them with a sense of fear and loss of control of their own life. I never wanted these outcomes for my mother, but at some point, I had to decide because it was for her safety and the safety of others on the road.

I also worried about her health because she was losing weight. So, I brought even more groceries, especially the foods she liked. Often, too, I went to her home to eat with her—or coax her to eat a little more.

My health declined. I had stress, acid reflux, and lack of sleep, worrying about her almost all the time and total frustration about getting no solutions despite my almost total dedication to finding some relief for her. Consequently, my depression and hopelessness increased. I discovered, too, that I had high cholesterol, and the acid reflux became so aggravated that it almost landed me in the hospital.

As a caregiver, I ignored most of these symptoms, except when they became too strong. And I forgot my feelings. My journal during the final year helped my stress and frustration at times, but it was never enough. I was exhausted. Many nights, I did not sleep, staying awake and thinking about methods and possible directions I could take and people I could call to find answers for my mother. Articles I'd read and people I'd talked to rolled around in my head, and I wanted to revisit these to uncover answers.

Sacrificing My Physical Fitness

I had no time to exercise or concentrate on my own health. I have always valued fitness and try to exercise in my little spare time because of my jobs and family. I'd been a personal trainer in college and an avid basketball player, so fitness was a priority . . . until I devoted myself to my mother.

My passion is playing basketball. I've had a group of friends for several years who meet at 9:00 a.m. every Sunday, and we forget life's responsibilities, have fun, and play. It takes me away mentally and physically for a few hours a week.

Fitness was a way to keep active and helped my well-being. I worked long days and even longer nights teaching. My only place to forget life and stress for a short time was exercise. I loved the gym, too, and was an avid runner. Exercise put my mind at ease and helped me emotionally and physically, but it was all put on hold because my mother was my priority, and her health was all that mattered to me.

I remember several weeks towards the end of Mom's life when I was all geared up to play. I had put on my long knee socks, laced up my size fifteen basketball sneakers, and then strapped on the protective gear. It takes a half hour to put on ankle braces and other equipment to prevent injury, but we play for the love of the game, stress relief, and exercise. As I was fastening on my gear around 8:00 a.m., Mom called. She was panicking due to her dementia, and I dropped everything and rushed over to comfort her. I never got to the court that day.

Such episodes recurred often, many times disrupting my sanity, health, and need for exercise. I do not regret going to help her, but my point here is how important it is, as a caregiver, to take care of your health. This aspect of caregiving is critical: take care of yourself first to better support your loved one. You are not sound mentally and physically if you do not care for yourself first. I did not follow my advice, and now it is a struggle, like having two people on your shoulders. One says to help the other person and the other says to help yourself. This is the one area I would have to revisit if I ever looked back on caring for my mother—doing a better job of self-care.

I would have loved for her to participate in exercise—and exercise has been found to help PD. We even built her a home gym in her house. She loved it, but when the disease progressed, she went from taking long walks to a stationary bike, to a walker, and finally to a wheelchair. And she lost hope. The progression was quick and unexpected, and we continued to try to find some way to slow the progression but were unable to. For the last seven days of her life, she was bedbound. I saw up close what Parkinson's can do to a person.

Expenses

We spent a tremendous amount of money on trying to cure Mom or at least curtail the disease. We also didn't have long-term insurance—who would have ever dreamed what would occur? Government help didn't exist, and we didn't know who to turn to. Towards the final year, we spent $12,000 a month for extra care alone because Mom needed constant supervision with her delusions and hallucinations from dementia.

Medical marijuana, too, was very expensive, and, because of our negative experience, we never even used most of it. We spent more money on her needs and wants and what we thought she would like. Each time we spent money, it did not help, and I was horrified. Our attempts failed again and again. I kept thinking of new ideas and spending more money—maybe believing that the more we spent, the better our chances of helping Mom. It was irrational, I know, but I was desperate and perhaps even superstitious.

We visited doctors, chiropractors, physical therapists, psychologists, psychiatrists, pain management doctors, and other specialists and agencies that supposedly would help my mother—or so many advertised they would. I wanted to believe them. I even purchased an alarm she could wear to call for emergency services, but she hated it, so I spent many hours trying to cancel it. We also hired numerous aide companies and a director to help me facilitate her care (which did not work).

You name it, I tried it. Maybe the next one . . . I would have traveled the world to find a cure, and my goal was to have no regrets but first to help cure Mom and have her with me for much, much longer. Like her, though, I often lost hope.

I bought anything my mother needed or wanted, with no questions—from a medical bed to a medical recliner to the new home supplied with ramps and accessible bathroom accessories. Although she never liked many items I bought to help her, I gave her choices and the best possible care. Television was essential to her, and I immediately took care of any adjustments or repairs. I knew when her favorite shows were on and taped them for her. I monitored her food intake—only healthy foods—and watched her diet for a long time. But eventually, when nothing was working, and she became sick of drinking bottles of Ensure, so I let her enjoy the food she liked for the rest of her life. I kept a list of the foods she liked, buying whatever she needed and wanted and stocking her kitchen. So,

I'd buy her favorites, healthy or not. One of her favorites was chocolate cake, and I often bought her two.

Despite all my efforts, it was difficult to pinpoint one aspect of helping Mom and then carry through. So many things were needed—medical supplies and equipment, food, and later aides. Bills piled up: all the medicines, groceries, banking, electricity, phone, heat, home upkeep and repairs, water, and then the fees for Reliance's private care. But I kept spending; no amount of money would stop me from getting the best care for Mom that we could find.

My Extreme Stress

It all came with a steep cost, though. I put Mom first, giving up any regularity in my own life to ensure hers would be as safe and steady as I could make it. As a result, my time with my wife and children was sporadic.

Something told me, too, that we didn't have a lot of time, so we needed to find ways to save Mom before it was too late. I thought I could always get back to my own needs once I solved her medical issues. Now, looking back, I'm sure this curtailment contributed to my troubles with my own health and lack of mental stability.

I even sought a therapist for myself because, at times, I felt so alone and struggled daily with all of Mom's problems. But I only went for three visits. It took too much time, and I thought they did not help me. At the time, I wish I had found a support group for caregivers of those diagnosed with Parkinson's, but I was not aware of any and, although I tried, could find none. Even though my wife was a steady and incredible support, I still had deep and dark times and didn't know who to turn to when all my efforts failed to save my mother.

Sometimes, I felt like I couldn't take any more. The mental stress of trying to help Mom daily, find new solutions, take her to the many appointments, and everything else involved in her care was a full-time job. I kept reminding myself that I would regret it if I didn't do *everything* I could for her. And I reminded myself, too, that she had cared for me unreservedly by giving birth and raising me. It tortured me later that when she passed at sixty-nine, she wouldn't enjoy retirement or see her grandkids grow up and start families of their own.

Mom's Thoughtful Planning

My mother was able to save money throughout her life, like planning for a trip or to enjoy her retirement. But the disease stripped her and our family of those imaginary plans. She was an incredible planner, though, and never wanted to be a burden on her family. Toward the final years, she planned everything she could. She didn't flinch from discussing tough topics with us and appointed me as her power of attorney. She hired a lawyer for her will and even took care of funeral expenses and planning. Of course, she didn't know all of these would be needed so quickly.

However, she was open and ready to prepare for the worst but hoped for the best. Anything and everything she did was for the benefit of others in case of the worst scenario. Sadly, it was all necessary and saved me a lot of additional stress, tears, and pain. It would have been far worse if she had ignored all the necessities and left them to me afterward.

I would have been thrown into chaos and even more pain and would have had to scramble at the last minute to attend to her affairs. Legal complications might have even blocked me from helping her. So much was avoided because she was incredibly thoughtful about these major, tough life decisions, even to the final days. I am thankful for all she did; her example is why I also have already planned for this in my life today.

Managing My Work

Despite Mom's careful planning, my work life suffered, too. I couldn't devote the time I wanted and needed to teach and advise my students, and I worried I would be fired from several of my adjunct teaching positions. I enjoyed helping my students but could not devote the time I'd previously dedicated to them because of the extraordinary amount of time I spent helping my mother.

I tried to figure out how to keep working. I succeeded in arranging my teaching schedule around helping my mother, which meant I worked virtually 24/7 instead of regular hours.

The Ultimate Challenge

My life was difficult to manage between Mom, family, and work. Initially, before caregiving, I felt like I was juggling a few small tasks, but when I assumed the primary caregiver role, I held an entire universe on my shoulders.

I have always been able to accomplish multiple tasks, but with another individual's life, it is much different. I did put Mom first, though, which challenged my relationships with friends, especially my wife and children. However, they were always supportive, and I knew they were by my side when I was in need.

Today, I walk by what would have been her home, and I'm overcome with sadness. I kept doubting my own decisions, even if she was still with us, because I couldn't handle the constant medical issues and her worsening hallucinations and delusions. Yet I keep wondering—if I had acted, made one more call, and found out about one more remedy, things may have been different. But, as the therapist said, eventually I knew I had to stop regretting and second-guessing myself because the disease got the best of us all. Finally, I came to realize that Parkinson's disease does not define a person, and being a caregiver is highly challenging. Still, it is worth every second of the love given and received.

The Male Caregiver

Maybe I was unusual in wanting to be my mother's primary caregiver. Generally, I have been told that women are the major caregivers—daughters, wives, cousins, and others. But I wanted to ensure Mom had the best, even though I later sought outside help. In this traditionally female role, more men are caregivers than is generally believed. From research for a speech I gave, I found that, compared to 19 percent fifteen years ago, today men comprise 45 percent of the caregiver population, one of three caregivers. This statistic surprised me because men often have a more challenging time with caregiving than women.

Why? Culturally, we're supposed to be stoic and not show or express emotion or vulnerability. This is where my journaling saved me. We approach things rationally and problem-solve. The goal was to fix the problem, as I attempted, with hours and hours of research into PD and contacting every professional I could find.

Men also don't usually get the emotional support they need. I am blessed to have Grether, who supported and understood me throughout. According to the article, more men work full-time *in addition to* caregiving—82 percent. I did, too, and felt great strain being pulled in all directions. As many male caregivers do, I hesitated to tell my boss, who is my dean at the university. But I eventually did and assured him I remained committed. Thankfully, he understood completely.

Male caregivers suffer from the same challenges as women—depression, exhaustion, stress, fear, sadness, and resentment. I certainly did—although not resentment. I could never resent Mom. And men get just as burnt out as women caregivers. I got very burnt out and didn't take care of myself enough. That "strong" male image prevailed until I became ill. Then, I was forced to look back at what I was doing. And admit I couldn't do it all alone. And ask for help.

With working at teaching and caring for Mom, spending so much time away from family hurt. But my mother's care was something I will always cherish and would have done without hesitation all over again. I am grateful for a strong wife and family. Their support was a critical component in my ability to care for my mother. My own support system was necessary, or I wouldn't have been much help to Mom.

Chapter 4: Steadfast Family Support: Partner

As I've said, family has always meant a great deal to me. My family supported me throughout my growing up and college years, and my wife helped me throughout this terrible journey.

In Brooklyn, when I was a child, we lived in a small apartment near Mom's mother, Grandma Pauline, who helped raise me. Her sister, Aunt Ellen, and her family lived nearby. Grandma Pauline dedicated her life to her children and pridefully raised them to be good, respectful, and honest. Pauline loved spending time with her family and paid much attention to Andrew and me. I could always count on her for support, care, and a hug.

She seemed to like me best and took me under her wing, teaching me important life lessons, good values, and respect, like she had with my mother. I have attempted to emulate Grandma Pauline with my own children.

Recently I found some old videos, which I cherish. One shows my birthday party when I was eight years old. Grandma Pauline, my other grandmother, Aunt Ellen, and her son were waving to the camera and smiling. I still remember the little horse they gave me; it had springs so you could ride as you jumped up and down. My mother always had beautiful birthday parties for me, inviting family and friends and baking a magnificent cake, which a video captured. Another video shows me sitting on her lap while we read cards and opened presents. I wore a silly hat and waved to the camera. Mom laughed, satisfied that her son was having the best birthday.

Grandma Pauline and Aunt Ellen moved to Florida in about 1988. As I said, in 1995, Mom moved us to Florida, wanting to be nearer to them. Grandma Pauline, Aunt Ellen, Uncle Scott, and Cousin Adam lived with her in Boca Raton, and we lived a block away. I was so happy to be reunited, remembering all our previous wonderful times in Brooklyn.

Sadly, Grandma Pauline passed suddenly on March 10, 1996. Because we had moved nearby in 1995, it felt like we did not have much time at all with her.

As anyone who has had an ill family member knows, everyone is unavoidably affected. A pall hangs in the background even during happy events, like birthdays, anniversaries, July 4 celebrations, and Sunday dinners. If the ill member can attend the events, the other members keep looking over to see how they are. From the moment of diagnosis, even with treatment, a nagging worry hangs in the back of everyone's mind that only worsens.

The effects on my family of my mother's Parkinson's were profound, and in this chapter, I quote Grether and the children directly. They can speak better than I about their memories of Mom and the disease progression. Perhaps their words will help readers with the reactions and recollections of their own families.

After our weekly Sunday dinners, Sharon loved to take the children to the backyard or living room and blow bubbles with them. Like Grandma Pauline, Mom wanted to be part of her grandchildren's lives.

The kids were delighted, but Grether and I watched anxiously from a kitchen window or around the corner as the illness progressed. Mom's hand progressively shook as she held the bubble wand. My heart sank, and Grether and I exchanged worried glances. Whenever I saw a new symptom, I resolved to do more for Mom, however I could. This thought was the only thing that would give me at least some peace of mind.

After dinner or any other event, I would withdraw and sit on the edge of our bed, my head in my hands. Grether would come over, sit beside me, and put her arm around my shoulder. "You're doing everything," she'd say, trying to soothe and reassure me. "You're doing even more than everything. And I'm here too." I'd hug her and almost cried.

Grether

Probably many husbands admire their wives, but I more than admire Grether—I marvel at her. She's raising our three beautiful children, has continued to study criminal justice at a Florida university, and is completing her undergraduate degree. She has participated in many charity events to raise awareness and funds for PD (see Chapter 11). And she supported me unequivocally in all the research, doctors' visits, and countless other things I did for Sharon. Grether suggested we build a big house and all live there, with a particular room for Mom.

How PD Affected Our Relationship

Most often, caring for a family member means neglecting the partner. The patient becomes all-consuming in time, emotions, and activities. And partners, despite their best efforts at generosity and understanding, may resent the time and attention the ill member takes.

A friend's wife was very ill with COVID, and my friend supervised her medications but couldn't handle being with her very much. He kept signing up for overtime at work and then went out with friends, staying late into the night. Once, I met him in the supermarket, and he looked awful. He admitted to me what he was doing and told me he and his wife had terrible fights because she thought he was having an affair. He assured her he wasn't, but my heart went out to him. I encouraged him to tell her the truth and go for help, but I don't know if he ever did.

Grether was a different kind of partner. It can't be denied that Mom's increasing symptoms and care took more and more of my time and attention. With my constantly seeing after her and my work, Grether and I had little time together. But Grether knew what Sharon meant to me, and we weathered everything together. Grether recalled, "I remember the first time I met Sharon. After you and I dated for a few weeks, it was time to meet her, and I was super nervous because I wanted to make a good impression. You always said only good things about Sharon, including that she was your best friend. So, we knew a lot about each other before our first meeting, but I was still nervous.

"I remember going into the Chinese restaurant, and you introduced me. Sharon was smiling—maybe she was a little nervous too, but as excited to get to know me as I was to know her. We hugged almost instantly. That was the beginning of a beautiful friendship between us. And she became my beloved mother-in-law."

Amazingly, after Mom got sick, Grether quickly came to terms with our division of duties. With her love for Sharon and respect for my relationship with her, Grether accepted what had to be done.

Grether said, "I do not feel the caregiving hugely affected my relationship with George. During Sharon's battle, the kids were tiny, and we were still going on with life as normally as possible, even though George was dealing with many things. George was handling a lot of Sharon's medical issues alone. I would take care of the kids. At the same time, our oldest son, Joshua, had medical problems, and I was helping him through some tough times, so this was difficult to manage. George would take care of Sharon but also work and keep the family going."

As a woman, Grether, too, understood what would make Sharon feel better. Grether would often tell me it was so important to help Mom continue to feel like an attractive woman—which she was. Mom confided in her how shocked and sad she was with her appearance. So Grether arranged for a hair stylist to visit Mom's home regularly to do her hair and technicians to give her manicures and pedicures. Some days, though, she was too sick and or hallucinating, and the appointments had to be canceled.

Mom would not leave the house in the final three to four years, so we decided to bring as many services as possible directly to her at home. I booked a massage therapist, but at a certain point, Mom was in too much pain to agree, and even this therapy became a problem. Grether bought her clothes from her favorite store. Grether loves fashion, and she had observed how Mom always chose a particular style of clothes. The fabrics were breathable, and the fashions were upbeat, with gemstones, and somewhat flashy (I always liked this).

My mother constantly asked us, "When will I feel better?" and "When will I get better?" We had no answers, which was heartbreaking for us. Grether felt my mother may not have understood Parkinson's disease because, for several years, she never discussed it, even when she had developed more symptoms. We did not know anything about the disease until the final years when I immersed myself in research and reached out everywhere I could think of.

As I said, Mom didn't bring up the disease and never mentioned it, so either she didn't understand it, knew nothing about it, denied it, or thought it wouldn't affect her as it did. Neither did we know it was so devastating. So, we could never plan or arrange specific things early, like exercises designed to help, or take steps in many areas I learned about. We were in a panic mode, which became the norm. We didn't know how long she would be in that state, how long she would live, or the answers to many other questions. Both Grether and I were extremely worried about the unknown of it all.

Nor had we ever heard of or were aware of the five stages of Parkinson's (see Chapter 2), and a large part of the reason we took over Mom's life was that she no longer could manage on her own. Grether, like me, is convinced that my mother did not want to be a burden to us, which is why she kept things from us, and we were so unaware. She loved us but did things her way. Even today, we question and still do not know why she never talked about Parkinson's. We wish she had shared more and that we had known earlier what Parkinson's is, what it does to a person, what stages it takes, and what stages she was in. Her secrecy, we still feel, added to the chaos and confusion about steps to take and possible treatments.

We never knew how far along she was, and by the time we found out, little was left to figure anything out or decide on a course of action. Also, research fifteen years ago was not as advanced as it is today, and, as I've said, Mom didn't share anything with us until the symptoms couldn't be ignored. And the doctors repeatedly told us that a person "doesn't die from Parkinson's." Because of this constant pronouncement, we had no reason to believe her health would decline so quickly and she would pass away so soon due to the disease. So Grether and I were immensely frustrated and worried as we saw the symptoms escalate, but not because of Mom. Instead, I was angry at the disease and the entire medical profession, which, I felt, had failed us.

Other Relatives

Other family members, understandably, may become worried about the PD patient. When our relatives heard about Sharon, many had a host of understandable questions and a lot of suggestions and ideas about how to care for her. Some also wanted to go to the doctors' visits with us, but that burdened me more. As I was consumed with caring for my mother, I found their demands for answers overwhelming. I had no answers, and I was dealing with nurses, aides, therapists, doctors, and, of course, my mother's needs.

Many times, due to her dementia, she didn't want to see anyone but me, either because of depression or the medications or because she didn't want anyone to see her increasing debilitation. I had to make excuses to the relatives, who kept pushing constantly. One family member wanted his art displayed on the walls of her house; he thought it would make her happy. My mother liked art, but, as with everything else, I was trying to maintain the house, and we were planning to sell it and move Mom in with my family. Putting holes in the walls and paying attention to things that didn't help Mom's health directly were not important to me. The only thing on my mind was my mother's health, trying to help make her comfortable and fighting her Parkinson's.

I couldn't be angry with the relatives, though. I knew that what seemed like intrusions and meddling came from their worry, love, and hope for her well-being. But it was all too much for me to handle. My only concern was my mother's health. Without her health, nothing else truly mattered. So, I let down the family members as best I could, thanking them and telling them that Grether and I were meeting Mom's needs, and I promised to keep them informed. I suggest the same for anyone in a similar situation.

Grether's Loyalty

I consider myself twice blessed—to have had Sharon as a mother and to have Grether as a wife. She has indeed been a support and partner at every stage. Many times, I felt completely alone and could always count on Grether. She was always on my side, there to support Sharon in whatever ways she could and to comfort, counsel, and support me. In her own words:

"We were there for her every step of the way to reassure her that things would get better and that she was not alone. However, the journey was just as much of a mystery to us as it was to her. I have experience with Parkinson's only through Sharon. I saw up close a lot of what she went through, even though she never really talked about Parkinson's much.

"It was in 2017 that Sharon started feeling worse daily when her symptoms showed more, and she could no longer hide them or brush them off. She needed to rely more on our help for tasks around her home, which she'd been used to doing independently. She stopped going to plays and restaurants, which she loved, because she had more trouble moving around. She had difficulty using her left arm, so we started eating more at home instead of at restaurants we liked. We always spent a lot of time together, and the time with us as a family helped her keep going.

Grether commented that the family's focus shifted from children, as is often the case, to Sharon and her care. "Caring for Sharon was the most significant thing that took up our time and attention. We all wanted her to be healthy and happy, and we wanted to do anything we could to help support and care for her—even the kids."

Nevertheless, Grether's focus was still on the children, and because of her almost total attention to them, I had the time to care for my mother. However, Grether and I observed with sinking hearts that even when Mom was with the kids—and she loved being with them—as time went on, she couldn't do much, like carry them, play with them, or read to them.

But we tried to take each day at a time. We knew we were in a bad mental state, a reactionary state because nothing definitive could be determined or planned from minute to minute. Grether was extremely worried about Mom's health, as was I, and despite all my outreach, we could only watch helplessly. We didn't have the luxury to take a step back and look at the bigger picture, but we wanted to spend as much time as possible together as a family. Because we were never told that my mother's disease would take her over entirely and end her life so quickly, we had no time to plan. It was all out of nowhere and too accelerated even to grasp. I felt mentally and physically out of breath. Before I knew it, I was thrown into something unimaginable, trying to claw my way out by any method or means to save her life.

Grether's Observations of George

A family member's death always affects everyone, even if some members hardly show it. I was devastated, and Grether noticed some significant changes in me. She said, "Sharon's passing did affect my relationship with George. It wasn't immediate because after Mom's passing in January 2020, the COVID crisis appeared, and we were in quarantine. Also, three months into COVID, our son Joshua was diagnosed with a tic disorder. But we were trying to spend more time together, which was nice and what we had wanted. But the COVID situation became overwhelming; with three kids at home, George was working full-time remotely, and we lived with the terrible uncertainty of when the quarantine would end. We were again in a reactionary state, having to respond to another crisis and not allowing ourselves to stop and properly grieve for Sharon and come to terms with, even accept, what had happened with her in recent years."

Grether continued, "George was very close with Sharon. Her not being here changed him. Not having her here left a void in his life, and he may still not have grieved fully. So, since 2020, he has sought to fill this void as a way of grieving. His method has been to advocate and raise awareness for Parkinson's research and cures. And he's done an amazing job—with the website, interviews, podcasts, speeches, presentations, and social media posts (see Appendices). I have accepted that he may not be as available to me emotionally as previously, and I believe in the causes as much as he and have joined him in the fight."

My Partner's Support and Participation

Grether is a beautiful example of a partner who wholeheartedly supports me and this cause. She got involved with awareness to find answers for Sharon because of her PD. Grether became part of a community that was going through the same thing our family did. I'll let her tell it:

"I've learned much about Parkinson's and the movements and organizations to combat it. I continue to support 'Moving Day' for the Parkinson's Foundation, a day for fundraising through walking, and a lot of money has been raised. So many more people are aware of it, too. During COVID, George and I did the virtual walk. We also participated in the American Parkinson's Disease Association 'Optimism' walks. I have participated in other activities too, such as the PushUps4Parkinson's and the 2024 half marathon in memory of Sharon through the Parkinson's Foundation. We have raised and donated about $15,000 to help programs and funding for a cure. And, of course, I fully support the website in memory of Sharon, which we started together.

"My goal is, like George's, to find a cure for Parkinson's. It is something everyone should be aware of, including younger people. With research and new findings, awareness is gaining a lot of ground. Individuals can detect specific symptoms or potential causes earlier, and discoveries can impact how the disease is treated. Knowledge and awareness are powerful, monumental, and essential. More people still need to be made aware. The more people who understand the disease, the more individuals will be knowledgeable and work towards a cure. Of course, this expanding awareness benefits all individuals diagnosed with Parkinson's, their relatives and friends, and everyone.

Grether also has excellent advice for relatives of people suffering from PD. "Stay connected to the people who love you and want to support you and others in similar situations. All these connections are vital for our emotional and mental well-being. Many people out there want to show love and support for you. It helps if you never go through something alone. Don't be afraid to ask for help and seek out connections."

Emotional Resources

I've never been very religious, although my grandparents and parents celebrated the major Jewish holidays. My grandmother was quite religious, and when I was young, we all met and said prayers. After my grandmother passed, my mother tried to keep up a few of the Jewish traditions. However, we were not that religious as far as attending the temple.

After Grandma Pauline died, my mother always lit a unique memorial candle for her on the anniversary of her passing, a *yahrzeit* candle. I've done the same with the family for Mom, and the candle burns for at least a day until it goes out. Whenever I catch a glimpse of it, I'm sad and joyful at the same time. I am unspeakably sorry, of course, that she's not with us, and yet I am so grateful for the time we all had together. I'm slowly coming to peace, too, with having done everything Grether and I could do for Mom within the limits of available knowledge and resources during the years of her illness.

With Mother, toward the end, I did feel that it would be helpful for a rabbi to visit with her and offer spiritual comfort.

But she was too sick for even one or two visits. Grether and I didn't seek therapy, though, because of the time constraints of caring for Mom. After she passed, as I said, I had a few appointments with an understanding man. But I didn't continue because of my work schedule. Perhaps if I had given it more of a chance, it would have helped. I believe therapy can help long-term if one devotes the necessary time and attention to it.

Today, though, I feel like I am in an odd spot. I do not have Parkinson's, and I am no longer a caregiver of someone living with Parkinson's. Instead, I often feel stuck alone—someone grieving the loss of a loved one who had Parkinson's. I've researched many support groups and found only ones focusing on those diagnosed and those currently caring for a loved one with PD, but nothing for someone in my situation. Yes, many grief support groups exist, but specific Parkinson's grief support groups are needed!

Instead, I've relied on my relationship with Grether. I've always had the confidence and comfort that Grether would support and help guide me to the correct answers and actions. She is by my side all the time. We talk about everything, and there was never a time we couldn't turn to each other. Nor have we ever had secrets. I value and respect her opinion; we've become a powerful team.

This description of our relationship may sound unbelievable, but it's true, and I count myself doubly blessed for having her.

What I've Learned About Sharing With Your Partner

Before Sharon became ill, I hadn't read any articles on how to handle a severe illness with your family. I learned, though, by living through it all. If you're interested or need to, see the resources in the appendices for family help and books for children.

The journey through Mom's Parkinson's has been a difficult one but one in which I've learned a great deal, not only about PD but about relating with my partner and children in the face of a debilitating illness. From the beginning, it was vitally important to talk with Grether. I've never been too open about my feelings, but I couldn't hide my intensifying worry from her. She saw it on my face anyway. And at every turn, she was completely willing to sit down, listen to me, and jump in with whatever was needed.

As I said, and I repeat with admiration and praise, Grether took over care of the children while I cared for Mom more and more. Every time I couldn't contain my frustration and anger at the disease, Grether listened quietly and didn't try to talk me out of my feelings. Her response was always, what can I do to help? So, these experiences have shown me what to recognize and do with your partner when a family member becomes seriously ill.

Realize the illness will change your primary relationship. As Mom's disease progressed, she became my major preoccupation. With my drive to seek help and glean as much knowledge as possible, I withdrew significant attention from Grether and the kids. It looked like I was willfully moving away from Grether, but this wasn't the case; I felt pulled by the PD.

You will have less time together. As I took on more, Grether and I had less and less time to be alone. We took what time we could—but it wasn't easy. She never held a grudge or complained. We managed to watch a few of our favorite shows and talk about them. But I often could not be with her because I was supporting my mother. Usually, I had to stop what we were doing and rush over to Mom's home to check on her because she would call me in a panic. Before Mom's health declined, we had scheduled a family trip to the Bahamas. We went, but from the time we left Florida to the day we got back home, she called me every hour to tell me she was worried about what the disease was doing to her.

Make time to talk about the situation. Grether was the first person I turned to for support and sharing during the horrible times and the rarely positive ones throughout my mother's illness. I asked for Grether's opinion and support on every step I took or contemplated acting on to help my mother. My mother had been that person I turned to before, but because of Parkinson's, she had no distance from the illness, of course, nor was she able to reason or give me the advice she always had. Parkinson's affected her mentally, physically, and emotionally.

Ignoring or minimizing circumstances is unrealistic and foolhardy. Grether encouraged me to talk and would always stop what she was doing and give me her full attention. My knowing we were in it together was itself a relief. Very quickly, we came to realize we could figure things out and make decisions together.

Communicate not only about the facts but about your feelings. I tried to hide them for a while, but it became too much. And when I unburdened to Grether, it was a great relief. During the most challenging times, she felt that I needed help and suggested therapy during and after Sharon passed.

Even now, four years later, Grether can see I am still grieving and has said she feels that with every year that goes by, I am showing even more signs of suffering. Recently, I was a guest on a podcast to discuss Parkinson's awareness. I am 6 foot 2 inches, 200 pounds, a cop since 2006, and have witnessed and been part of many challenging situations. Yet following the show, after talking about my mother, I walked into the office and started to sob. The conversation brought back haunting memories of the final year of Mom's Parkinson's disease and what it did and took from me. It took the mother-son bond and an irreplaceable love.

I am still grieving today and realize that my many concentrated activities and outreach on behalf of Parkinson's awareness and a cure are ways to sublimate my grief and keep Mom's memory alive. I feel comforted, though, knowing it is all for a good cause.

Remind each other that you *can* cope with this and will do your absolute best. I was never much for a Pollyanna attitude, but I fully needed to remain positive despite all the setbacks. Grether saw the importance of this outlook and maintained it with me.

Honor each other's needs. Your and your partner's needs become even more critical because so much of your energy is given to the ill family member. So, ask what you need and encourage your partner to do the same. Grether knew I was an exercise addict, and so at different times, she arranged to take care of Sharon while I went to the gym. I realized, too, that Grether herself needed outlets. So, I encouraged her to go running, which was her hobby. I also told her to continue to pursue her academic and professional goals and not feel guilty about doing so.

I encouraged Grether to take care of herself in other ways, like having dinner with her sister Elizabeth. And I sent Grether to the spa with Elizabeth and my mother-in-law Joaquina. They loved to get away and forget everything else for a short time. Even though I missed Grether when we were apart, I knew she needed time away.

Your relationship may become stronger. Adversity always brings people together, even among strangers. It is no different with family, especially with close and special members. Although Mom's outcome wasn't what we had worked for and hoped for, Grether and I became much closer and even more vital as a couple. We became more confident that we could make it through anything life could throw at us.

We discovered talents, abilities, and reserves in each other we hadn't known. For example, when I had to rush my mother to the hospital, Grether would be right there to support me. She understood the intricacies of the medications and scheduling with so many doctors. And I was delighted at her wholehearted participation in all my causes. She has often told me how much she admires my perseverance for Mom and dedication to her memory. Grether recognizes my leadership role, and yes, we have occasional disagreements, but we resolve them with a foundation of love, trust, and mutual dependence.

* * * * * *

Grether and I rely on each other, understand each other, and have become true partners through the whole experience. Now I know we're a *team* and can face anything. In grappling with and getting through something like a relative's Parkinson's, it is supremely important to have someone you can trust and confide in and know will always be by your side.

During Mom's illness, Grether was a steadfast support, and she continues to be. I have experienced her constancy and love—for me, the children, and Mom's memory. If anything is to be gained from this awful experience, it is that we have developed increased respect and love for each other and has grown immeasurably closer. This is true for our children as well.

Chapter 5: Steadfast Family Support: Children

When a family member has a horrible disease like Parkinson's, your children can be a burden or a welcome tonic. Through their play and carefree mindsets, they can add to the onerous responsibilities or become a respite from the constant worries. We were blessed that our children loved Mom and loved to be with her, as she did with them.

Caring for the Children

Grether once again took the major responsibility for our children during Mom's illness and made their worlds as normal as possible. She never felt put upon, though. "I do not feel like it was ever a burden," she said. At the onset, Brooke, Sharon's first grandchild, was eight years old, Joshua was six, and Eli was three and didn't know how to talk. Grether said, "Their world was small, so I had to ensure they could continue normally, grow, learn, and adjust to life."

Brooke and Joshua were especially close to Sharon. Sharon loved to read to all three and always gave them puzzles and balloons. Grether observed, "I know she dreamed of being there for them as they grew up. But the disease stopped her from that opportunity."

Grether also knew how important the family routines were. Even when Sharon needed a full-time caretaker, Grether noted, "We all kept Sunday get-togethers intact. Sharon loved watching the kids play outside together and always remembered to bring bubble kits or coloring books for them every weekend, no matter how she felt. I will always treasure those Sundays we spent together. It was a foundation piece to our family unit."

The Children: Brooke

The children, inevitably, were affected too. As the oldest, Brooke was most touched. When she was eleven, she remembered this. "I was very sad. I was seven and eight years old, and at first, I did not notice a lot, except that Grandma Sharon could not do things as much with our family. I remember having her around less after she became very sick." She continued, "Many times, I was unsure why my father was so busy. I thought he was at work. Later, he told me he had to spend more time with my grandmother to help her."

Brooke was always concerned about her grandmother. "I went to school during the weekdays but always asked how she was doing. I would see my grandmother mostly on weekends when the entire family went over to her house, or she came to ours to eat lunch or dinner and spend time with her." Brooke may have noticed that Grandma Sharon couldn't cut food, but Brooke was also too young to fully recognize the decline of Mom's health. When Brooke saw my mother hug a pillow and thought it was hers, she giggled. I've noticed she responds with laughter to things that make her uncomfortable. Still today, one of the most difficult things in my life was trying to explain my mother's disease to Brooke.

Later, Brooke remembered more: "I remember when Grandma Sharon became sick. I knew she was sick because Daddy told me. We were all very sad. But I liked the ladies that took care of her. I remember she used to come over on Sundays and watch me play. She always brought me gifts.

"Grandma Sharon was so nice; we went to restaurants together too. I think I looked like her when she was younger, and I like that because it makes me remember her. I miss her so much. It is good that Daddy cares and has started TogetherForSharon® to remember her."

Reflecting on what the experience taught her, Brooke was thoughtful. "We need more awareness because kids may not have the information. We can be confused and scared when we see things. We need to understand Parkinson's and know what our loved ones may be going through. I join my family on Parkinson's [charity] walks and wish we had a cure, because I miss her a lot."

Brooke's words brought back a very painful memory for me. It was the day we came home from Mom's funeral in 2020. I will never forget walking into the kitchen after the funeral and seeing Grether hugging Brooke, who was sobbing uncontrollably. It had hit her: she loved her grandmother and realized she would never see her again. Even writing about this brings me pain. I think Brooke realized then that this wonderful person she loved would never be able to play with her any longer or share anything again.

Being so young at the time, Brooke didn't know much about Parkinson's, but as she's grown older, she has become tremendously interested, especially seeing me advocate for awareness and hope for a cure with my many activities. She has gained much understanding and now goes with us to charity events. Of our children, Brooke felt the loss the hardest, maybe because she was the first grandchild. At the time, she was young and emotionally immature, but her responses were wholly understandable and, with the closeness she felt with Mom, to be expected.

The Children: Joshua and Eli

Joshua was six and Eli was three when Sharon became ill. I realize now more than ever that my children were affected by Mom's long illness. How could they not be? No matter how young, children see, hear, and understand much more than we realize. But I don't think they remember much. Joshua certainly loved my Mom and spent a lot of time with her. He may have wondered why the visits stopped, but he didn't ask me or Grether.

Eli was still a toddler, so I wondered if he even remembered my mother. But this is part of why I advocate and share her memories— to ensure he never forgets. We also played videos and looked at pictures, like those of our wedding, which had videos of some of the most beautiful memories that Mom, Grether, and I had ever had together.

Mom and the Children

Grether and I tried to be sensitive to the children's needs, curiosity, disbelief, and occasional horror. We included them in all the Sunday dinners, even when Sharon became more incapacitated. We took them to visit her at her home and the hospital. We spoke about her often to them and recalled happy memories so they wouldn't forget her, how devoted she was to them, and how much she loved them.

We would take the kids to Mom's house, and she would bring out all my old childhood toys for the boys to play with. Brooke was fascinated with Mom's piano and would immediately sit down and start "playing." (Because of her ongoing interest, we later gave her professional lessons.) The entire family would gather and sing on birthdays and major holidays. Mom also attended Brooke's preschool graduation, which was a treat for them both.

On one special day, I recall Grether arranging a beautiful sixth birthday spa party for Brooke. Brooke and her little friends gathered, gave each other manicures, and took turns styling their hair. They even had a fashion show. But Mom missed the day because she was too sick. She would have enjoyed it greatly. For me, the day was very rough. Mom called that morning, saying she wanted to attend but was feeling too sick. I felt terrible that I had to choose whether to go to the party or be with her. There were many times like this, troubling and difficult choices I had to make. On this day, I stayed for Brooke's special day for a little while and then rushed over to Mom's.

I knew the children felt neglected, especially by me, because Mom took up almost all my spare time. I had hardly any time to dedicate to the kids and see them grow because Mom needed me. But Grether devoted herself to them when she wasn't helping me. I gave them the time and attention I could and was involved with them when possible. I helped them with schoolwork, played with them, and spent time teaching them life lessons. But because my mind was so taken up with my mother, I felt I should have been there more for them. Often, Grether had to take Joshua to doctors' appointments, and I couldn't join them because I was busy taking my mother to other various medical professionals. The other two children were left on their own for short periods, although my mother-in-law Joaquina (a saint) lived with us and helped care for the children.

I located all our old childhood photos, and often Mom and I would reminisce about the better days pre-Parkinson's disease. Although I took many videos and photos of Mom's final year to remember her, now I never share them because the disease cruelly obscured how amazing and what a beautiful person she had always been. Parkinson's strips a person of both internal and external beauty.

What I've Learned About Sharing With Your Children

The principles are similar to those of sharing with a partner for sharing the serious illness of a family member with your children.

Talk with your partner about approaches, amounts of information, and times to talk with the children—each separately or together. Grether focused on keeping life as normal as possible for the kids, and I fully agreed. We didn't place any major expectations on them and let them be just kids. They showed their love naturally—to us and Grandma Sharon. Our focus was on living as normally as possible.

Don't hide the illness from the children. They know; they intuit; they read the signs—body language, silences, hushed tones, intonations. You're doing them more harm than good by trying to keep the illness from them (eroding their trust in you, for one thing). We never tiptoed around Mom's condition in the children's presence like, for example, when we had to be referred to a new medication or doctor.

Eli's youth protected him. He played and ran around without any fear and was too young to realize my mother had a disease or anything about its complexities. I often worry today that he was so young, three years old, he may never remember her.

I recently asked him how much he remembered about Grandma Sharon. He said he didn't remember her, which I find immeasurably sad. He will never have her love, interest, encouragement, and respect for the major events in his life and what he may become. Of course, in some measure, this lack goes for the other grandchildren, too.

But I often show them videos and photos of Grandma Sharon and hope my kids will keep her memory alive. They may even explore my website in Mom's memory with all its resources for conquering PD, TogetherForSharon®.

I think Mom could have had at least ten years or more and would have seen Eli grow up, but Parkinson's stole a grandmother away from her grandchild. As I reflect, I am sickened to see how many things Parkinson's disease can take away and how many secondary victims it can affect—not only the individual diagnosed but also the caretakers, family members, and friends, and probably so many more I'm not even aware of.

Take the time for the children. Sit them down. Tell them you have an important thing to talk about with them. My youngest, Eli, has a shorter attention span than the other children, which is normal for a small child, and he always wants to get back to his play. His favorite thing is having us all be together to watch him play. I wrote down the few things I wanted to tell him about Grandma Sharon: how much she loved him, how she enjoyed coloring with him, and how when she held him as a baby and looked at him, her eyes lit up and sparkled with love. I told him he changed her life for the better, and even though he may not have understood everything I said, he grinned and giggled.

Make your explanations age appropriate. For very young kids, simple sentences and main ideas are the best. Answer their questions directly without additional explanations. Older children may be interested in more details and even research.

Allow them to pursue what they need to. For each of our children, we explained what was happening with my mother, and we did so differently because of their ages and capacity for understanding. Eli, for example, was so young he understood only the most basic concepts.

Don't be upset if they don't seem to respond. They may need time to get used to the idea and take it in. Even Brooke quickly got back on her phone.

Answer their questions unflinchingly. Children want to be able to ask their questions safely and without reprimand. Tell them what you know and don't know. Grether and I told our children that the doctors kept searching for cures.

Share your feelings with them. By being transparent, you're not only letting them in but also being a role model for authentic feelings. They may ask, "Daddy, are you sad?" Tell them the truth about your feelings.

Tell them the truth about the situation. To do this is very difficult, and experts' opinions vary. Do we describe the appalling details? The children may see, in PD, the relative's hands shaking and may hear the delusions.

I described these briefly to the kids but not in detail, so they knew what to expect when they saw Grandma Sharon on Sundays. If they ask, do we tell them the relative will likely die? We don't know, and miracles have happened. I found it was better to say I didn't know than make a dire pronouncement. And I was being truthful—I kept up hope as I continued to seek out research and every possibility for a cure.

Involve them. When I told the children, Brooke immediately said, "What can I do?" I gave her simple tasks, like helping Sharon with her food at the table and reading to her. And I told them all, "Tell Grandma you love her and hug her."

Grether suggested we bring the kids over to see Sharon as much as possible. When we did, it was the only time my mother seemed to smile. If we could make her more comfortable, we did and had the children surround her with toys and laughter.

We wanted to steal her mind away from the disease, even for a short time daily. I knew we all would fully support the effort. Some days, though, Mom was so sick she couldn't walk and didn't want to be seen. She felt so sad, depressed, and ashamed because she was losing weight, getting skinny, and having involuntary movements. She didn't want to scare the kids, she said. And happily, she was never violent, as some PD sufferers are. So, we had no concerns for the children's safety.

In a way, in their innocence, children do not see the outcomes of Parkinson's. They just see their grandmother. I told Mom that, no matter what, we all loved and supported her, including her grandkids, and we would bring them to see her, however, she might appear.

* * * * * *

Children want to feel they are a part of the family and the effort to help. Doing what they can gives them a sense of control over the situation, helps them cope, and gives them tender memories of their relative.

Grether often told the children, "We are going to visit Grandma Sharon." Mom made an entire playroom in her house so they could play. She would go into the playroom and watch them play, smiling and laughing at their antics. I treasure this wholly positive memory, one of the few embedded in my mind forever.

My children, too, helped Mom enjoy the little time she had remaining. They were a joy to her and got to know their grandmother, at least somewhat. The love and laughter they shared are priceless; my heart was lifted every time I witnessed it. I am so grateful that they all had at least this time with each other. If anything is to be gained from the awful experience, our family has gained more respect and love for each other and grown immeasurably closer.

But even with the wonderful support of Grether and the joys of my children, I still had all the tasks for my mother, keeping up my job, giving my family what attention I could, and getting little sleep. Eventually, I was overwhelmed and burned out. So, I felt forced to hire helpers.

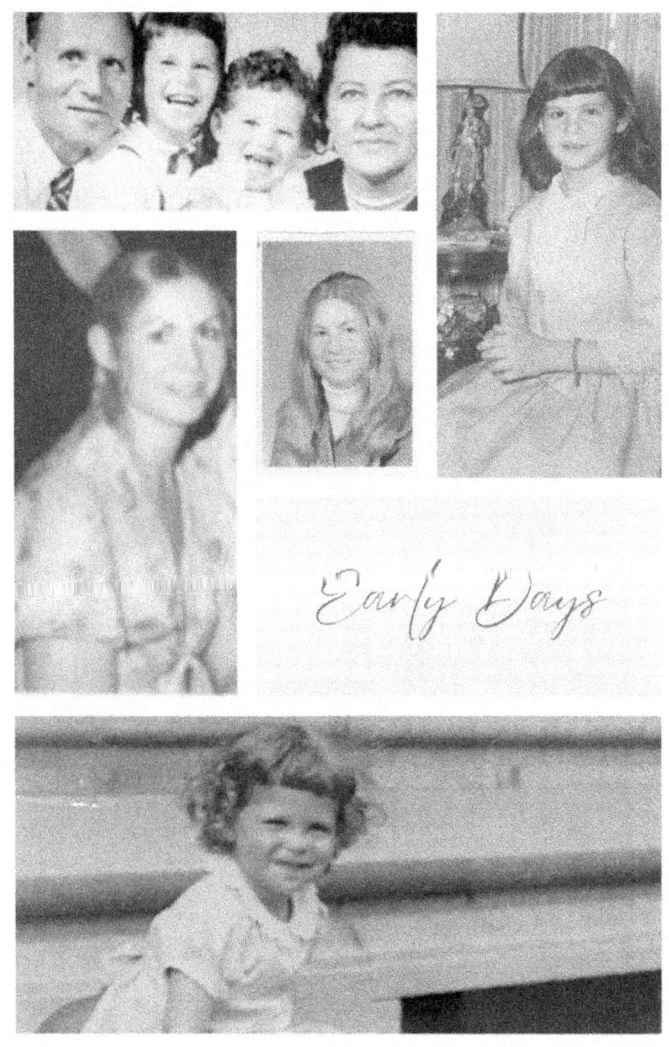

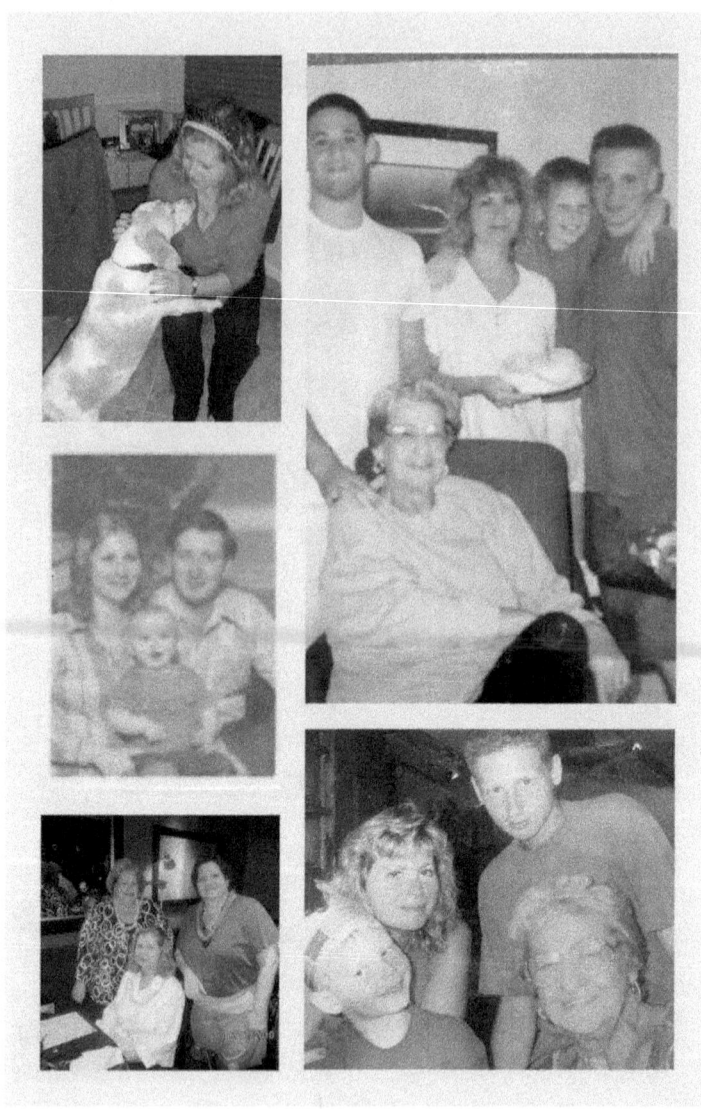

Family

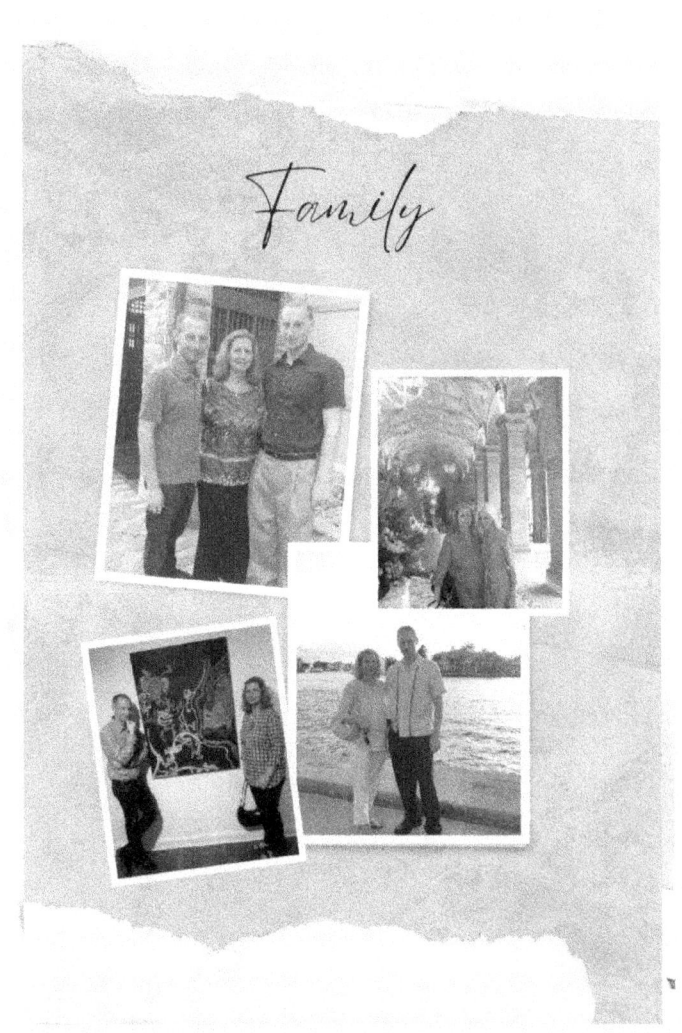

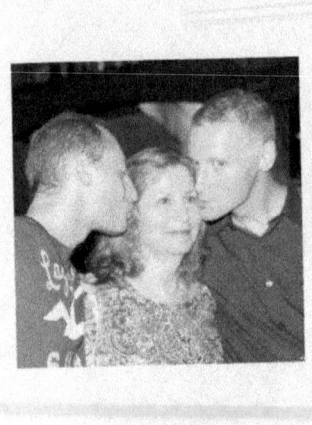
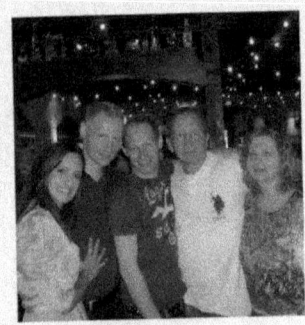
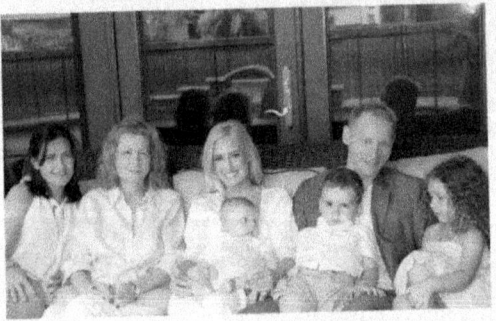

Forever in our hearts

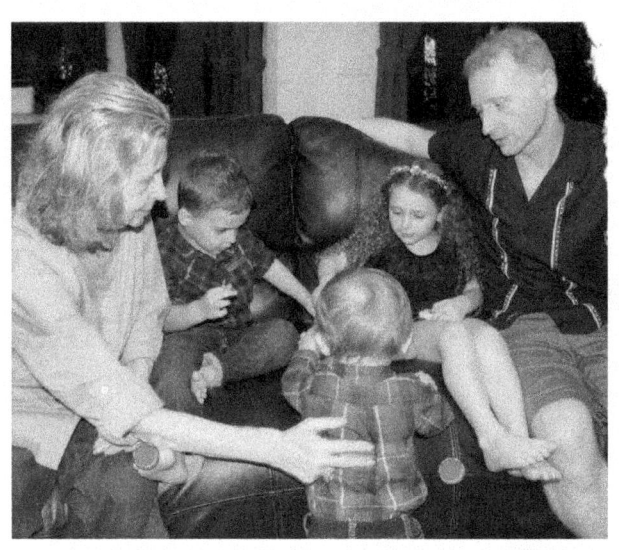
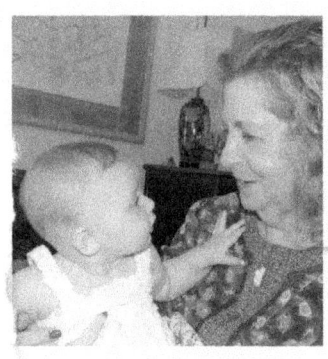
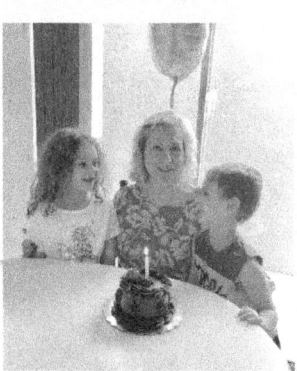

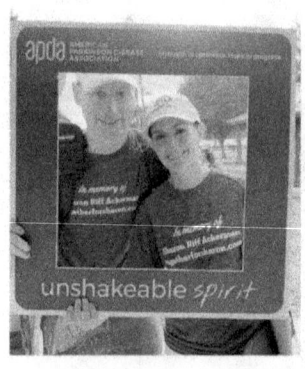
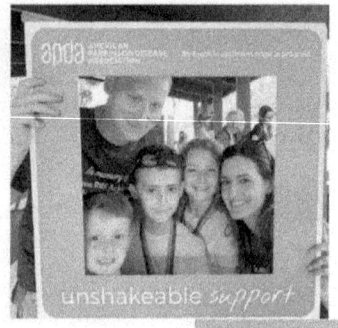
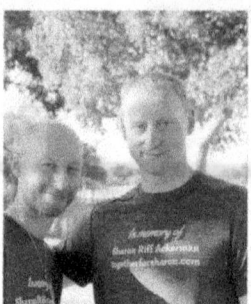

Advocacy

IN MEMORY OF MOM

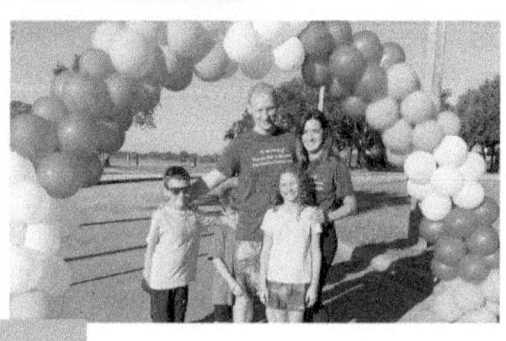

Chapter 6: Trying to Find Good Aides and Caretakers

I wish this chapter were more complimentary to aides and caretakers. I'm sure there are good agencies and good aides, who, as a woman on the supermarket line once remarked to me, are in it "with their heart." But this was not our experience until very close to the end. Not only did Mom suffer; we all did. As my mother's health declined, I was already strained with my pursuits and, even with Grether's unwavering help, I found I couldn't take care of Mom full-time. We had to employ aides and caretakers.

We hired aides for the final four years, from February 2016 to January 1, 2020, the day she passed. Finding a decent company took four years, seven companies, and over ninety-five aides.

I did a lot of research. I asked people I knew for referrals, mined the Internet and television ads, and even hired someone to help me locate a company. South Florida is known for many of these types of services because we have a large elderly population. So, originally, I thought it wouldn't be too hard to find a good agency. Except for the last one, the aides we employed, I'm sorry to say, were much less than good. (I've purposely used the word "care*takers*" in this chapter because we found most of them takers rather than givers.)

They were inattentive and not trained to help with Parkinson's patients. In addition to my worries about Mom's Parkinson's and dementia, I felt the acute strain of the aides who were supposed to help her and lighten her burden and mine.

I wrote the following journal entries primarily for catharsis but also to chronicle my search for satisfactory aides. The entries are also cautions to readers who may need them. Sometimes I wrote more than once a day because writing was a release that helped me cope, and I didn't feel right about constantly unburdening myself to Grether. Other days, I had no time or was too exhausted to write, so the dates are irregular.

June 11, 2019

8:00 a.m.: My mother calls very upset and cries that I shouldn't forget her and take her out of her place and to my house. She believes people are harming her. I calm her down, but these calls are constant, repetitive, and almost round the clock. She says the nighttime aide is mean but likes the daytime aide. Yesterday, she loved the nighttime aide but hated the daytime aid.

She will not hang up and begs me again to pick her up so she can come and live with me. She is upset at her family and keeps repeating, "Please don't forget me." Then she refers to a man harming her in the past when she was younger; I explain that no one will harm her now. She's worried about the doctor's visit today, and I assure her she will be okay. She finally hangs up.

But she is also afraid of the aides, and most of the time, I am not sure if she is telling the truth, or the companies are bad. I don't think she knows either.

I am not sure how much more I can handle on my own. Now, I have a headache and feel sick after her call. We installed video cameras to watch over her because we caught one aide neglecting her. I was up all night worrying about her, and when I looked at the camera, I saw nothing but the aide caring for her. Finding the right aides to fit all our needs has also been a struggle. This is getting harder for her and me every day.

Yesterday, I went to visit my mother. We arranged for a hair and nail stylist to surprise her at her home. Even that turned out to be a challenge. When I started to pay the stylist, we saw my mother, as in the past, hugging a towel because of dementia and calling it my daughter's name. This was not only embarrassing but disheartening and sad, and I was sure the stylist wouldn't want to return.

I'm taking care of everything and reassuring Mother constantly, supervising the aides, case managers, doctors, and so much more, and I still feel like I am failing. I don't want to have the kids around either because I don't want them to see her with mental issues. They just do not understand. She also wouldn't want her grandkids to see her in this state.

I am burnt out and have no one to turn to for help because we have no cure. I am not medically or emotionally able to care for her, but I am trying so hard. We are paying for full-time two-shift aides and barely making the bills.

June 20, 2019

Mom wakes up every day saying "Sorry" and "Mommy, Mommy." She continues to plead, "Please, Mom," talking to her own mother. But, her mother, my Grandmother Pauline, passed away decades ago. Delusions and hallucinations are taking over.

Mom is angry, flailing her arms and screaming, "I must pee, right now!" She runs from her bed, and no one can control her. She says the aides hurt her, and I keep checking the cameras to make sure they don't. But she is more confused and scared daily and no longer understands where she is. She twists off the bed and falls.

The aide tries to control her and raises her voice, screaming. This aide who's there now is rude and angry and should not be caring for individuals with Parkinson's.

Mother needs care and patience. This is not working out, and I have no one to turn to for help or guidance.

Despite my paying a lot of money for help, she is not in good hands, and it seems many of these aide companies are scams. They claim professionalism and nursing services, but none of the employees are nurses—I checked credentials—or professionals. The fees are over $12,000 per month just for the aides because Mom needs 24/7 care. We started with aides in February of this year and have gone through three already. I will be firing the fourth soon.

I won't stop until we find the right aides and a company that cares. There must be a company and employees who aren't in it just for the money and taking advantage of desperate people in need. I know in my heart there have got to be decent people who really want to help—somewhere.

June 25, 2019

Every day, something is not right. The current aide company is not very good at communication, making it tough to provide my mother's care. She thinks the new aide is a murderer and says she was in prison. The dementia is worse daily. Mom also yells, curses, and blames me for her Parkinson's but calls me her father and the names of others like my father, so I know she's not rational. This disease takes the mind and is killing us all. Mom has been the most positive, caring, loving, and incredible person I have ever met. But the disease is taking all this away, as well as her hope. It's horrifying to watch every day and getting worse and worse. . . I am lost.

The company seems to send ten to fifteen different aides, so we are all confused. As usual, I am unsure what to do next. I run back and forth ten times a day from my mother's home to ours to soothe her, and I am burning out.

July 14, 2019

My family and I went to the Bahamas on a trip planned a year ago. There were nonstop calls by nurses and aides, and it was tough to enjoy anything. We cut the trip short and came back early. Mom's health was the same, and we still had to deal with everything. I am so thankful for Grether and my children, my mother-in-law Joaquina, and my sister-in-law Elizabeth.

They helped Mom while we were away and are the only individuals who keep me sane and at least somewhat positive.

July 17, 2019

Mother was sick and missed every doctor's appointment this week. The medicines are not right, and we can't get her to see doctors because she misses appointments and is too sick today. But she agreed to go to the hospital to have her mental state checked and see the psychiatrist and the neurologist. We started getting her ready at 2:00 p.m., and I paid the case manager to help. She gets $125.00 an hour (almost unbelievable) and came to the house. With her help, my mother would have had a chance to get the medicines under control. The case manager took Mom to the hospital and then left. But my mother decided not to stay and went home with my brother Andrew.

I spent over eight hours today on her care-related issues and have paid thousands. We are right back at the same spot as months ago, nowhere with medicines. And I just fired a fourth agency. I feel like I'm wasting time and money. And my dean at the college called me in and said if I didn't fulfill my teaching duties, he would have to let me go. But I don't have the time, and worse, I haven't seen my kids in weeks.

This can't continue much longer. I don't know what to do and feel alone. We're trying everything and anything to help Mom, but we can't find the right assistance. She's not the only one losing hope; I am, too, even though I don't want her to see it.

I have had to plan the medical times, days, and appointments and get her back and forth to the doctors. It is all very hard, and my head is spinning. She needs round-the-clock care shifts, which are not easy to find or afford.

Again, I would do it all again, but I wish she never had to go through this; she had been so independent and did not like anyone helping her or aides living with her. That was the toughest part for someone like her—to lose that independence and privacy due to a disease.

July 20, 2019

I woke up thinking that today might be relaxing. I was hoping for a mental break because I couldn't handle the stress, with so much I had to do for Mom daily and the time constraints. I love helping her, but I have reached my breaking point. At 10:00 a.m., Mom called and then five times during the next hour. She complained that she was being hurt by the aides and how horrible life is. I tried to be positive to her, but this was nearly impossible.

How many years will this continue? I feel horrible about not being able to find a cure or any resolution for her. Now, there's not much more I can do, and I know it. Parkinson's disease is horrible for everyone, and I feel completely lost and alone trying to help Mom.

July 26, 2019

The aides don't know how to deal with her. Right after the change of aides today at 8:00 a.m., she begged to go to the bathroom. The two who came on were talking and ignoring her. She sits in the wheelchair and says she must go to the bathroom, but they don't pay any attention to her and continue to ignore her. One empties the trash, and the other watches. They just leave her sitting as she calls out for help. She rolls around in the wheelchair on her own, unattended, and a few minutes ago, threw a tissue at the aides to get their attention. But one yells, "You must wait. I'm doing something."

At 8:10, I observe the aides screaming at her to sit down. They are frustrated and unable to do what we need, nor are they trained at all for this job. Their behavior is unacceptable. This is not the service I am looking for. I will let them go today, but finding a caring person has been impossible, and I won't rest until we do.

The case manager is nice but cannot answer the issues, and the doctors are even worse. This continues . . .

July 26, 2019, Later On

Today, I spent over four hours interviewing new aides. I went through over sixteen companies to find one that could assist us and have some basic understanding of Parkinson's patients. I am drained and not feeling confident at all. I hope with my whole heart that this works out.

However, we hired and fired seven other companies. I had to yell, plea, and beg the assigned aides to help my mother, and all of them were terrible. One even brought Mom to her own home without my permission. That move could have been disastrous.

August 4, 2019

The aide called today and said that Mother thinks I am her dad, which is so sad. She is not aware of where she is and thinks someone is trying to take her away. I just breathe and try to cope with it. Some days are good, and some are bad. Although the other aides have been terrible, I am thankful for Reliance, whose aides and nurses are there 24/7 for our family. There are not many options, though; either just allow the episodes or medicate. That is all I have learned in all the years trying to take care of her part-time, and now full-time.

August 7, 2019

The aide called me this morning, and I spoke to her and my mother. I asked Gerry, Mom's best friend, to please discuss with the nurse what she notices when others are not around. Gerry said that once everyone leaves (including the Reliance nurse), Mom becomes much more confused, upset, unable to walk, and constantly needs to use the bathroom. Also, my mother told me this morning that she fell twice yesterday, yet Gerry and the current aide said she had not fallen.

August 8, 2019

My mother was in very bad health the entire day yesterday as Parkinson's crept up. Two nurses came out from Reliance, but nothing worked. I need to figure out something more. Mom called me one hundred times throughout the day, and I felt helpless. She also left me ten frightening voicemails.

Mother's dementia is worse as well. She thought someone was going to kill her, then thought the nurse was taking her away to a facility. She kept fighting with them verbally, which was not all her fault. It is this horrible disease.

Thankfully, my mother never showed signs of violence, which is often a symptom of the disease. Violence would have just added another major problematic behavior. One time, though, when I was not present, the aide explained that Mom was so frustrated due to the disease that she threw a light fixture against a wall, and it broke. I do know Mom was very frustrated and often blamed Parkinson's for ruining all our lives. But I was still right there by her side, no matter what the disease would bring or how tough it would be to tackle the everyday constant side effects and devastating progression that continued to increase.

I am not sure what else to do, but I can't go on as is. I am absolutely lost again . . . . It is painful and heartbreaking.

August 8, 2019, Later

I had to call Reliance to send nurses three times today. Either Mom is over drugged or took nothing. In both cases she becomes overly anxious and cannot sit still or stop moving. There doesn't seem to be a middle ground. She is safe with aides watching every minute of every day and night, but this is no way to live. Every time we went to the ER, they pronounced her healthy. They know as little as the aides. Baffling, horrendous disease.

I wrote this today to the dean at my school by way of explanation for my lateness and absences: "I don't think I told you, but my mother has Parkinson's disease, and it has been a horrible few months. I have been trying everything to assist her, from aides costing over $12,000 a month to the hospice helping me with nurses. But there is really no hope with Parkinson's, and it is draining to see a loved one, especially my mother, deteriorate. I cannot do anything to fix it. The only positive outlet that keeps me going is teaching, and I am so grateful for you and the students. The only way I can keep my head up is through this. Thanks for listening." He responded that he understood and would give me some leeway. I resolved to continue fulfilling my teaching duties, even with everything else.

August 9, 2019

I fired yet another nursing company and hired another, the fifth. The aides had left the room and Mom fell. It was another horrible day, and I still must deal with the kids, work, and home duties.

What I Learned From Interviewing and Hiring Aides

The difficulty of finding a good aide company or individual aide to help care for Mom led me to make a list of errors, troubling behaviors, and cautions to keep in mind when interviewing the companies and aides. Prior to finding the final excellent aides from Reliance, I still cannot believe that in my four years of searching and incessant interviewing, I had to remind the so-called professionals of some of these areas.

We do not want Mom to remain only in her bedroom permanently. So, daytime aides, take her outside to the patio, help her walk, help her do things she no longer can do herself.

Never leave Mom alone; she fell once when she was left alone.

Please remember to follow the medicine pill box instructions strictly, and if anything runs out, notify me or the nurse immediately. Some did not follow the correct medicines, doses, or schedules, all of which are life-threatening.

Please be pleasant and supportive.

Don't wear perfume.

Keep areas clean.

Don't yell at Mom. She has Parkinson's and dementia and may need extra care.

BE ABLE to understand Parkinson's disease.

Understand dementia.

Understand fibromyalgia.

Understand the possible hallucinations and delusions that come with PD.

Communicate with Mom and with me. Communication is critical.

NEVER SAY "HOSPICE." The word tremendously depressed and upset my mother.

Grether understands the role caretakers can play. She said, "Caretakers have a huge impact because they are the individual's primary ally. The caretaker is the person they are with most of the time, and the person they can vent to and be honest with, even more than doctors. The caretaker becomes their whole world. Hopefully, everyone is lucky to have someone to lean on during the good or bad times. It is a journey, and the ill person needs someone to support them and give them strength to help them through."

We finally found a company in which the aides understood and supported Mom.

Chapter 7: Finally, Great Caregiving

In this chapter, I share my experiences with the aides of the new company, CaringComforters, and I intersperse my journal entries with reports the aides sent me and occasionally my posts on social media. I finally found and used support groups on social media for caregivers of loved ones with Parkinson's. We all try to help each other cope and understand what others may have been going through. And I have made lifelong friends.

My entries and the aides' reports chronicle my mother's horrific, inevitable decline, and yet the aides' messages show their sense of responsibility, acute observations, and caring. Anyone in my situation should look for these qualities when hiring a caregiver for a loved one.

August 12, 2019

Finally, I found another aide company, CaringComforters, although regretfully so late, toward Mom's final three months. But there were conflicts with Reliance. The aides assigned by Reliance, Aleena, Lurene, and Betsy. were excellent because they really understood Mom and cared about her. We all considered them like family.

September 7, 2019

It is sad and almost unbelievable to spend thousands of dollars a week mainly for Mom to have gloves, diapers, wipes, and bed pads. Just gets more depressing daily. No one should have to live like this. It keeps getting worse.

September 14, 2019

Mom may have had a mini stroke. Every time I think it can't get worse, it does. Six months ago, she was okay, but now, daily, she seems to decline more due to this horrible disease. She refuses to get a brain scan and now cannot do almost anything without assistance. It's horrifying to see my mother and best friend continually degenerating.

I posted the following on my Facebook and shared it with the support groups I had joined. "I know you all have similar stories, and talking and hearing stories means the world, but I feel so alone and helpless most days."

She must have known too how serious her condition was because she started saying goodbye to everyone. But she can hardly talk and only whispers. Most of the time, I am unsure of what she is saying. Soon she may not be able to eat anymore, and I fear the worst will be coming before long. Just don't know how to do this. I avoid posting pictures on Facebook, but I am unsure how to explain what I see or even believe this experience is occurring. I feel that every day I am losing my best friend a little more and more . . . .

She never had a chance or the time to plan for this, but then again, no one ever can. The disease creeps up out of nowhere and is unimaginable. I try to keep my spirits up by thinking about the earlier years before ever having to learn about this disease. Wish it didn't exist . . . .

September 16, 2019

For me and my family, the word for the month is "Hopelessness."

September 18, 2019

Today has been horrible. She called, screaming, and cursing that she was in pain. Then I got the nurse to go to her house, and she refused to get help and yelled, "I have a terminal disease and want to die." What can I do? I have a bad headache and am just burnt out trying to find solutions. I have no idea where else to look anymore. Reliance changed the medicine,

Methadone, to 5 mg day, 5 mg night. Doesn't seem to make a difference.

September 20, 2019

The saddest thought is I cannot spend as much time as I should or would like to with my mother herself because I am taking care of her bills, aides, housing, food, and anything else that comes up to ensure she is taken care of in the best possible way. It's very costly, though. Mom spent all her retirement savings, and we have provided and continue to provide a great deal of money to help her with everything. No one else is helping financially at all. The irony is that by taking care of everything for her, I can spend less time with her. It is the worst inner battle for me daily.

September 23, 2019

I saw my mother again today. She had slept continuously for a few days, and I don't know if she even knew I was there. Just hope she's not in pain. I'll do anything and everything in my power to be with her and take care of her—forever. We've now moved her in the brand-new home next to ours. She only smiles lately when the kids are screaming, hugging, and kissing her. Family is the only cure that Parkinson's won't ever defeat!

September 24, 2019

Mom can barely speak. We have aides and pay tremendous fees to ensure her safety with Reliance nursing care day and night. We have video cameras, we visit daily, and I call five to ten times a day, but she does not know we are there and, most days, doesn't answer the phone. I swore I would never put her in a care institution and will not. We settled her into the new home, and we rent old Broadway shows and movies for her. But she barely looks at them and only seems happy when the kids are with her, shrieking, squealing, and playing in front of her.

In just six months, she went from a cane to no mobility at all. We got her a bed that moves up and down and a wheelchair, but she hates it.

Either she has no medicine and is hallucinating and acting out through anxiety or is highly medicated and unable to talk.

There is no middle ground. The disease is winning the battle, and the worst thought is that this could continue for a decade. I only hope she is no longer in pain. The progression of this horrible disease has crushed us all and is torturing us daily.

September 25, 2019

Saw Mom today with the kids, and she was 100 percent fine and happy. After we left, the nurse reported to me that Mom lost it, couldn't understand where she was, didn't know where she was going to live, and was delusional. Whenever she is with us, she is fine. This disease is horribly fascinating and terrible, frustrating, and baffling.

September 26, 2019

Yesterday, we went to visit Mom, and from 5:00 to 7:00 in the evening, she was an angel, and the kids all had fun. The second we left, she called me and was frantic, asking me to drive to her old New York house in Mill Basin, New York. This is where we lived over thirty years ago. She was obviously delusional and hallucinating. She threatened to call the police if we didn't take her to New York.

Seems that when she is around only the kids and me, she is fine. When anyone else is there, she is incredibly bad. The aides need to be more in control of the phone at night and provide relaxing drugs or give her drugs to calm her agitation any time she is like this. This episode could have been prevented, and it's not safe for her. That is why I have aides. I must tell the supervisor of the aide company to help me straighten that out.

September 28, 2019

Today, I realized I won't be able to speak to my mother on the phone any longer. We used to talk eight to ten times a day and night and did so for almost my entire life, even in my adolescence. I knew she would always be there for me, and I could count on her. So, when she couldn't speak or respond anymore, it was heartbreaking.

At this point, she is too weak to speak. Most days, when she's awake, she hallucinates and is unsure where she is, where she lives, or what day it is. Otherwise, she is resting or sleeping. Last night, again, she asked when I could drive her to Mill

Basin. When I tried to explain, she got very upset and did not understand where she was or who anyone was. So, depressing. I feel like I've lost my best friend.

September 30, 2019

There are three September birthdays, and we celebrated them today for Mom (sixty-nine), Andrew, my brother (thirty), and Brooke (seven). Mom came over to my house for several hours today and was doing great! It was the first day she'd been able to come to our home and stay without pain or other PD complications, as if she'd never been sick. Today may have been the best day she has had in years, and it was so amazing to spend time together. One of the best days of my life!

I am so grateful and cherish every second seeing everyone smiling, laughing, reminiscing, and enjoying being together. I am grateful and thankful for today. I'll try not to forget this memory because I know tough times will be ahead.

October 7, 2019

The aide texted me that the nurse was at Mom's house and said she would call me. This was the nurse's report: "Sharon is not herself today. I had to keep moving around with her because she would not stay in one spot too long. She is very confused and has bad hallucinations. She keeps talking about things I have no clue about, saying I'm stopping her from saying goodbye to her kids."

October 18, 2019

I received a text from the aide Betsy from Reliance and then asked her how Mom was doing today. She answered, "That's a hard question to answer. Sharon's health is so up and down. She is very depressed on top of her Parkinson's. All morning, she talked to herself about things I'm not sure happened. We will be in the bathroom for a while. She must have an enema. Zahara, the RN, said to do the enema now and give her the morphine and Lorazepam so she can relax and hopefully sleep. She also suggested that if I cannot do it by myself, I should call for a nurse to come out and help."

Mom's overall health seems to be getting worse every day.

October 25, 2019

I think Aleena, one of the other Reliance nurses, noticed too that Mom was declining rapidly in health. The quick, unanticipated decline is making her more and more depressed.

Aleena reported, "She talks a lot about death today in the morning. Asks about her grandma, her Mom, and Dad. Parkinson can cause dementia. I'm seeing signs of that. Sharon became more and more confused and hallucinating. But now, there is a big change in her mobility. I must literally pick her up all day today to transfer her. I'm sitting with her now at the table, and she seems a lot calmer here. She just said it feels like it's all cut up inside her mouth. I see a little whiteness on her bottom lip when I look. Maybe she had bit her lips, but no bleeding or redness to it."

October 27, 2019

Another text from aide Aleena: "This is not to ruin your Sunday, but I wasn't sure if you saw your Mom yesterday. I had to wake her up to get washed up and take meds. She didn't use the bathroom on her own like she usually does. She's becoming more now on the incontinent side, going in the pull-ups. Which is a form of diapers. Mom is very weak today, making it difficult to lift her by myself because no one else is there to assist me. I might have to keep putting her in bed a little after each meal and change her in bed. The aide on last night said she might not be able to come back and is quitting because of the lifting."

October 29, 2019

My mother seems to be in the worst stage of the disease. In just eight months, her health has declined horribly, and she cannot speak now. Each time I think it can't get worse, it does. Speech and movement have been the latest and final straw.

My not being able to communicate or hear her voice has been another final shock from this horrific disease. She is also now bedbound. She can no longer speak on the phone or in person when I visit daily. The worst, and a paradox, is that her health is good otherwise, despite the loss of speech and ability to stand or move. It is torture. No other word could express what she and we are going through daily. It's so ironic—and unfathomable: Mom had no other major health issues except PD, which is causing dystonia, dementia, and stomach problems.

November 3, 2019

I normally talk about my mother's Parkinson's disease and how horrible the progression is. Even though I take pictures and film videos, I only posted photos of when she was younger. I made videos and took photos for myself to remember her. I think, too, that if the scientific community ever needed them for research, I would assist. But I avoid posting them because it is so tough.

However, tonight, we visited, and I didn't record anything but couldn't get the picture out of my mind of the state she's in. She is doing worse, even when worse isn't possible. It is difficult for the kids to see and hear. I'm burnt out and frustrated at the lack of support in the medical field and almost all aide companies.

Trying to keep on the best we can. According to the nurse, she is healthy. However, she does not look or act physically healthy and is not mentally healthy. So, either this disease is a curse because it downgrades an individual's entire life from mentally to physically, or medically people just haven't studied it at all or enough. I'm so thankful for the Facebook friends and support groups but am frustrated.

November 6, 2019

Report from Aleena: "It's the middle of the week, and here's an update of what I have noticed this week so far. The crying is happening more. I asked the nurse about it, and she said they can't control that, and Sharon will have those moments on and off. Yesterday late afternoon, I noticed Sharon's left fingers staying close together. With all Parkinson's clients I have worked for, I have seen it happen because of loss of mobility or arthritis. I gave her that blue ball [for exercise] to keep the fingers from closing. I think it's called trigger finger. Have a good night until tomorrow."

November 7, 2019

Report from aide Betsy: "In the bathroom, just got done with her teeth. At the table for breakfast, Sharon had a breakdown moment, with crying, and she did the same thing earlier. This nonstop crying about Paul [Mom's husband, my father]. She seems better now but has bad hallucinations and confusion every day. The only time she doesn't is when she is sleeping. I love it when the kids come over because she changes in a quick second. I know it's hard for you to decide whether to bring the kids over when Mom is not doing well at that moment. Touch base with me when they are thinking of coming, and I'll let you know how she's doing then."

November 7, 2019, Later On

From aide Lurene: "I am sure you know Sharon's mobility has decreased to a point where she can't stand. She is talking to herself more. Some of the things are subconscious, and some are conscious. Sharon seems to feel she has been hurt in the past, physically and emotionally. She tends to remember this at times, and that causes her to be depressed. Early this morning, I gave her a bed bath, took her to the kitchen, and made her some coffee. She began to cry and talk about your Dad, saying she tried to forgive him. I felt for her. I hugged her and told her everything was OK."

November 9, 2019

Mom refuses to take her medicines now and is tortured daily. She wants her life to end. This is horrible . . . 24/7 HELL. And it doesn't even summarize what is going on here daily.

November 14, 2019

Tonight, we visited my mother. The pain—to see her tortured by this disease night and day. She has lost the ability to move. Most of the time, she is crying. She hardly speaks, and when she does, I cannot make out what she is saying. And she needs help eating. What is so baffling is that, medically, she is healthy. I wonder what they base this on and how they can say it. I think Mom's condition got worse when she started to lose hope. She used to ask me when she would get better and that she wanted to be there for her granddaughter Brooke's wedding someday. But she stopped asking, as if she knew that because of this disease, she would never get that opportunity.

Seven months ago, she was walking. If the disease is moving this rapidly, I do not think we will have much more time together. The entire situation is heartbreaking and more frustrating than anything I have ever encountered in my life. I share all this to hope and pray for a cure someday for others. It seems to be too late for us.

November 16, 2019

I have a continual headache and migraine all day and night from this whole situation, and neither the situation nor the headache is going away.

November 18, 2019

From aide Aleena: "Good evening. So far, Sharon's week has been the same: still crying on and off, confused, hallucinating, fearful, and her speech most days not clear. Her mobility is no longer there, not even to stand, but she asks to use the bathroom. I feel terrible, but I cannot take her when I'm alone. I'm unable to hold her up and pull her pants down or up or the pullup. I'm not sure how we can work around that, but I will take the opportunity to bring her to the bathroom when I have someone there to help."

November 20, 2019

From aide Lurene: "Morning, George. Sharon slept well last night. However, her talking to herself has increased. She is also having muscle contractions, which do occur with certain stages of Parkinson's. Her posture is also altered because of it, and I think that's the reason she is always crying from spinal pains. Overall, I think even though she is going through physical and mental changes, she is still strong based on her vitals. Have a blessed day."

November 25, 2019

I had to write to the president of Reliance tonight to ask at what point, when you see your loved one has no quality of life at all, do they step in to do something more to help? It was a horrific way to see my mother crying in pain daily and nightly.

And I have no idea how to help or when this would all end for her and us.

Dizzy from all of it. This disease was at Stage 1 for ten years, and now Stage 5. The worst of it is that it is torture for myself and my entire family, but I am grateful to have the support, kind wishes, and words of others. Trying to just keep going on for her.

Seeing the decline for the last seven months live and through video and pictures is something I don't want anyone else to see or go through ever in their lives. Hug your loved ones tight every chance you get and enjoy all the time together. Cherish every minute because those are the best moments in life! Sometimes, we let them go by too quickly without realizing in the moment how precious they are.

These are my strongest words, realizing the preciousness of love and at a time when these words are deeply needed.

November 28, 2019

This was the first Thanksgiving with Mom bedbound. She cannot stay awake, so she

can't celebrate. Her seat was empty this holiday, and I did not want to celebrate without her. And without her, it would never be the same again. She always sat to my right; we shared stories, laughed, argued, and enjoyed every second we were together.

I spent an hour writing to politicians about states with the right to die with dignity laws. Florida is not one of them, and it's awful. She would never want to be like this. She specifically told me that, and it is in her will. I never heard from the damn president of the hospice.

December 4, 2019

From aide Aleena: "Good evening. I always give my updates on Wednesdays. Sharon did well for most of the day. She did have two crying moments earlier today about Paul. But they did not last long, and she did not complain of pain until around 6:40. Then she became agitated even though she got all her meds that are required for pain, with agitation and

Parkinson's medication. She still seems a little agitated but will calm down soon."

December 12, 2019

I'm very grateful for these aides from Reliance. They are so conscientious and keep me informed.

From aide Lurene: "Just a little update while I sit here because Sharon is still sleeping. I woke her up to eat, but she refused to. I will tell the other aide to try again when she's fully up. I will only get Sharon out of bed once a day, and honestly, sometimes she doesn't want to because I have to lift her. The nurse practitioner recommended using a Hoyer lift [a mechanical device for a single caretaker to lift a patient]. Or when two people are around, we can get her up to prevent us from hurting our backs. Other than that, it's been pretty quiet. She only had one agitated, hallucinating, and fearful moment after 12:00 p.m. and kept complaining that she wanted to get back into bed."

December 14, 2019

Grether and I went to visit Mom, but the muscles in her face were dropping, and she couldn't enunciate words. She started to whisper. I was sickened, and Grether was very sad. We didn't know if it was a stroke, if the disease had taken over, or if she would ever recover. We added these questions to the long list of confused and startling things that continue to show up.

December 17, 2019

Stage 5 of Parkinson's is the worst thing I have seen in my lifetime. I don't even know how to keep going, seeing my mother like she is. And worst is not knowing how long this will continue for her. She is either on medications, sleeping, or crying in pain all the time. The hospice people are with her all day and all night every day and every night.

She has no quality of life and cannot really make sense due to loss of the ability to use her mind and the fibromyalgia, with pain throughout her body. A year ago, she was not that bad, and she asked me to promise never to let her live like she is now.

In the throes of all this, I kept posting on Facebook PD support groups to connect and show my gratitude. "Thanks for listening and for your time, as always. You helped me cope with this nightmare. I hope yours isn't as terrible."

One year ago, she was walking with a cane and could live. Today, she is bedbound with round-the-clock aides who are tremendously costly. But I'd give my last cent to find a cure. I avoid posting videos and pictures because they are so horrible to look at and comprehend. Seeing the changes is crushing every day.

December 20, 2019

Update from nurse Zahara: "Not on oxygen anymore for aspirations in breathing. It was only for a few days. A foley [catheter to drain urine] will be put in her bladder. She is not eating or asking for water. We think she is not coming off crisis care this time and to let go of the aides."

December 24, 2019, A Day Before Christmas

Mom is resting today. She does not wake up much any longer or communicate. She is still with us but not as responsive, and the nurse says her resting and medicines help her stay in peace. But I suspect this may be close to her final time with us. As long as she is not in pain, I am thankful.

I just feel drained and speechless. I see no end in sight to this. A nurse told me this state could go on for decades, or a day. My mother has no quality of life whatsoever. So, I sit, wait, and constantly ask myself: Is there something else I missed? Then I look and look and hope an answer will come. It's been over ten years since she was not good, but she was able to live. But from March of 2019 to now, she just deteriorated, and it's been painful and heartbreaking. I don't want to think about what is next from here.

Florida does not have laws regarding dying with dignity. However, we allow our animals more dignity than human beings (see Appendices).

December 25, 2019, Christmas

Sucks . . . just sitting and waiting for Mom to take her last breath. Horrifying. Every time a nurse sends me a text, my heart stops. Torture.

Nothing else to say . . .

Chapter 8: The Final Week

I don't look forward to the holidays anymore. Ever since Mom passed on January 1, 2020, the weeks and days leading up to New Year's trigger all the horrible memories and growing hopelessness. My body and mind both remember, and in the years after her passing, I've gotten sick almost like clockwork right around Christmas. I know it's not fair to Grether or the children, but all I want to do is stay in bed. And that question keeps nagging me: What more, what else could I have done to improve her quality of life and extend her living?

December 25-30, 2019

This past week, she has not been able to function. Reliance, the hospice, has taken over, and the nurses feel she has only days or hours left. We are entering new avenues that were not given much attention in Florida—end-of-life and Parkinson's disease. The law did not include Parkinson's disease when people seek palliative care or end-of-life care. The death with dignity laws are woefully insufficient.

We still sit and wait . . . She has been breathing, and for six days now, with no food or water. Impossible. Still with us and so strong.

She is unable to speak, open her eyes, or eat. She is likely in pain around the clock, and the nurses can only keep giving her morphine. It is excruciating to see her like this and torture for us all.

December 31, 2019

Mom loved music, and her favorite artist was Kenny G. In fact, in 2023, on what would have been her seventy-third birthday, Kenny G. sent me a video clip with a birthday message in which he played for her.

Kenny G's video reminded me that we used what could be called music therapy for Mom only at the end. She changed my life and always worked hard to ensure that my brother and I had great upbringings. I remember during college, one year there was a major New York snowstorm. It was so bad that school had to be canceled for a whole week. My mother noticed I was bored or needed a new hobby, so she suggested I take guitar lessons. Mom got me a guitar and lessons, and all these years I have played for relaxation and fun. I never thought I would ever be able to learn how to play guitar. But because of her care, love, support, and faith in me, I learned and have played ever since. Music has been a means of therapy for me, and it has changed my life and the lives of those around me. I am incredibly grateful to her now for the lessons.

I would grab the guitar on many holidays and play for the family. Whether on holidays or when I was trying to learn a new song, my mother always put up with the loud music. Sometimes, it was soft rock, and others, with my wide-ranging taste, from Sinatra to Elvis to Dave Matthews. I always had a passion for all types of music. I never dreamed that I would have needed the guitar to have one final connection with my mother as well.

It was a week before she passed. Earlier, we had had a music therapist come to visit her a few times. If we could take her mind off Parkinson's even for a few moments a week, it was well worth it. She had been too sick some days, but there were others when she truly enjoyed it. She sang along with the music therapist and smiled. Little did I know that at the beginning of the last week of Mom's life, I would step in and play one last song for her.

When I was a child, as I've said, my mother often took me to Broadway in New York City. She loved musicals, and we saw *Cats*, among many other shows. One of her favorite songs from the play was "Memory." By the last week of Mom's battle with Parkinson's, she had become fragile, frail, and bedbound. She couldn't speak but did try to whisper. She couldn't move much, and I could tell there was no coming back. But I wanted to care for her still and give her one more moment that she could cherish forever.

When the music therapist came, I asked him if I could sit in on that day, and I brought my acoustic guitar that mirrored the one my mother had first bought for me. The therapist and I agreed that we would play "Memory" from *Cats* for her. Little did I know it would be the final time.

So, we played, and the music therapist sang. I was able to videotape us but did not film Mom because she was so sick. I know she wouldn't want to be remembered for how she was doing at that point. We played for only a few minutes, but it felt like an eternity because I knew it would make Mom comfortable, happy, and smiling despite whatever hold Parkinson's had on her and us all.

For that magic moment, we played like our lives depended on it. It was one of the most beautiful moments in my life. When the music therapist and I finished the song, we looked at one another and then turned to Mom. She smiled and told me, in very halting and hard-formed words, that she "loved it" and "thank you." I was so appreciative of her reaction that I just let out a deep breath. I never knew if it was my relief that she could forget the disease for a few moments or my acute pain, because it was obvious she was still suffering. Then I realized those were the last words she ever said.

The few days after this, she remained bedbound still but had a heartbeat. She no longer spoke and no longer could open her eyes. Parkinson's had utterly taken over, and for the next few days, Grether and I and other family members gathered around Mom and just cried. We waited and remembered, not knowing how long or when or what time or day she could leave. It was devastating . . . .

Looking back today, I am so grateful for those times of happiness, the culmination of an incredible person's beautiful life. From the moment I was brought into this world, my mother was my hero and always will be. There is nothing like this bond, nor will there ever be another like what we had, the irrevocable bond between a mother and son. Parkinson's disease will never take away that bond or defeat all the unique and beautiful memories. Her memory will live on forever through all those readings of this journey, and I will never stop advocating for Parkinson's awareness and hope for a cure for her memory. I swear by it.

* * * * * *

We have no celebrations this year. I just bought the *yahrzeit* memorial candle to light every year to remember and celebrate Mom's life. Even though, as I said earlier, I've never been very religious, I remembered that Mom always lit a *yahrzeit* candle for my grandmother, Pauline. I want to show my children how to remember Mom and never forget her. She lived to see her grandkids grow up somewhat and looked forward to spending time together with them.

I may want to say a little prayer for her, too.

We had prepared, as hard as it was, with her will and funeral arrangements, but I couldn't face any of that yet.

The final night I couldn't help reflecting on her history of mobility and independence. My mother was one of the most independent people I have ever known, on her own most of her life. She was healthy her entire life until her Parkinson's diagnosis.

Mom was always excited to drive her favorite Lexus car, visit with her best friends, or go where she wanted and when she wanted. Parkinson's ended all her independence.

Even before PD took such a ferocious hold, one of the most challenging days in my life was in 1997, when I had to explain to Mom that, with the PD symptoms, I couldn't let her drive her favorite car anymore. It wasn't an easy decision, and I dreaded telling her. But I knew that if she continued driving, she would become a danger to herself and others.

So, one night after dinner, I sat her down and said I had something important to tell her. I couldn't find any kind words, so I just blurted them out. "You can't drive anymore, Mom." She didn't say anything but looked stunned and then outraged.

The only thing a person has is their independence; when it is taken from them, they lose hope. And worse, when that independence is made with an announcement from their child, it is even more heartbreaking.

Slowly, her health deteriorated, and by 1997, she stopped driving and went from taking long walks to losing the ability to walk without assistance. She learned that, despite her fear and anxiety, she would need to adopt alternative means to live and get around. The simplest acts and pleasures most of us take for granted, like walking to answer a phone, were no more.

In 1997, Mom was forced to learn how to use a cane. It was not a natural method to walk, but it was necessary. She lost her balance but adapted to the new life with a cane.

A year later, in 1998, she had to move to a walker. My children were fascinated with the walker and thought it was a toy. But to Mom, it was something she had never dreamed she would be forced to use. It helped with stability but was bulky and almost became an appendage. She could no longer go anywhere without it.

By 1999, she was forced to use a wheelchair. Her health had declined so rapidly that we were in shock, and we kept trying to determine any ways we could think of and researched incessantly to combat the disease. I battled daily, as I've said, to research a cure, consult doctors, or discover any methods we may have overlooked to help her. I kept feeling like a failure, and each day something new and more frightening surfaced with her health that made me sick to my stomach and affected my health. I suffered, too—from stress, poor sleep, missing work, and not seeing my family.

But strangely and miraculously, despite the escalating setbacks, until the final three years, she lived a relatively normal life. I will never forget Mom pre-Parkinson's for the firm, independent woman she continued to be.

My Letter to Mom

On September 24, 2017, my mother was rushed to the emergency room for the first time after an attempt at a cure through the university failed when she joined a trial study for Parkinson's.

I decided to write her a letter during that emergency room visit. When we got home, I gave it to her, and her face lit up. I am grateful that at least she was able to read it. She loved it and always kept it with her until the end.

To my best friend of my entire life, forty-two years, my Mom:

You brought me and my brother up to be hardworking, honest individuals with integrity, care, and passion for helping others. Following your example, I have dedicated my own life to embodying and extending the values you taught me, like good nature, commitment, and care for others. You instilled these values in me, and I live by them with everyone I meet.

I remember that anytime I finished something important, like an accomplishment, you were the first person I wanted to share the experiences with because you were always there to listen, praise me, and give me the best advice. From joining a fraternity to changing my major fifty times in college to law school graduation to reminding me to call you at the end of a police shift to the birth of my children, you listened eagerly and supported me. Or, as importantly, to share my day with them. You were always there for me.

You taught me to cherish life and enjoy every day and always reminded me that all one can do is their best. For many years, I didn't understand what that meant. But today, looking back, I discovered it means to try as much as you can in life, and it is okay to fail. It also means never giving up on the passion and desire to be positive and understand your path in life.

You are not only my mother but my sister, teacher, mentor, best friend, and so much more.

You are the most positive person I have ever come to know. You always looked at the good side, even when you reminisced about some unpleasant events, despite my face turning bright red. Like when you told everyone at parties of forty people, "George, do you remember when you were a kid, and you climbed onto your bureau, and it collapsed, and we ran in and only saw your head under it?" Or when I got hold of baby power as a kid—you can imagine what happened next and what my room looked like.

These were only two of the thousands of reminders I had daily of how you recalled and cherished our memories together. Even in the last years, you still loved telling stories, but now, thinking about it, what I think you were truly doing was making sure I passed on the memories we shared to my kids and their kids. I will never forget or let those memories be forgotten, and they will be part of us all and will live on forever.

You are my role model, inspiration, and the first person I always rushed to share my days with. And you always have been throughout my lifetime. As my mother, you have been the light in my life and have taught me to be the person I am today.

I am grateful for you, Mom, and I feel the world will always be a better place because of you.

January 1, 2020

Mom just passed away—6:05 p.m., January 1, 2020.
She can finally have peace.
And I am in shock . . .
Memorial, January 3, 2020, at Mom's Funeral

Two days after Mom passed, we held her funeral in Boynton Beach, Florida. I gave the following Memorial at her home in Boca Raton. We hadn't known when her passing would occur, and facing it now was a struggle and absolute torture. So many, many relatives and friends attended that I was crying just looking at them all.

"Thank you," I said, "for joining us today and taking the time to support my family and me. As many of you know, I have gone through this battle with and for my mother for a very long time, trying to do everything I could to help her. I only realized my helplessness several months ago when I realized my best friend wasn't going to be able to be there as she wanted to be due to this disease.

"Early in my relationship with Grether, I always joked with my mother and Grether, my fiancée at the time, that every time we went on incredible adventures like horseback riding or riding in a hot-air balloon, the second we got into the car on the way home I *had* to call Mom to tell her every detail. And it wasn't only because of Grether. I was always excited to share my life with Mom, even up to ten times a day.

"A few months ago, she stopped recognizing me on the phone and then couldn't answer, and I felt lost without her. That is when I knew this disease and the torture it causes families was going to get even worse. It went downhill every day after this.

"She had Parkinson's disease actively for over a decade, but it never started to affect her primary life abilities significantly until around 2014. She could still function and spend her favorite day of the week, Sundays, with us in the backyard, blowing bubbles with her grandkids, eating the best meals we could find, arguing with everyone about where to eat or what to eat. I will sorely miss those funny arguments.

"I am grateful beyond words to her caregivers who took care not only of my mother but me as well, and those fantastic aides became family. I was able to turn to them during the darkest hours for my mother and me, especially during the past several months. They were there for me unflaggingly when I had no one left to turn to discuss my mother's health. I was constantly on the phone or with them in person, frantic and hopeless, and they always came through.

"Sharon was only sixty-nine years old, with a lifetime ahead to see her grandkids grow and share more memories with us all. Toward the end, she spoke only of her grandchildren and how much she loved them, even when they would all make a lot of noise simultaneously for no apparent reason when we were all together. She always had so much love to give.

"Near the end, we were just a few days away from the family moving in together in a new house. I deeply regret not completing it, as I dreamt of us all being under one roof and that she could finish her life together with me."

* * * * * *

At the Memorial, I also read that letter I had written to her in 2017. Even then, I knew, sadly, I would read it one day without her, and today was the day that I had dreaded for years.

Then I continued, addressing everyone: "To all of you here today and those who couldn't make it, I am grateful to you all for your support, care, time, concern, and love. I won't let Sharon's memory ever be forgotten, and I will never forget the love she showed us all. Through my efforts and my wife's and children's, she will always be remembered for the incredible person she was and always will be.

"Finally, Sharon Riff Ackerman will join my grandmother and her mother Pauline, her father George, my grandparents, and be at peace. I am hopeful and confident in that.

"Thank you, and I love you all as Sharon did.

"I only wish I could have done more. Although it is tragically too late for us, a cure for Parkinson's disease is desperately needed. I pledge to do my all to advocate for this result."

Chapter 9: Family and Friends Remember Sharon

On the third anniversary of Sharon's death, I wanted to do something more and asked her family and friends to write short remembrances of her. The response was overwhelming, and it made me appreciate her, who she was, and what she was even more.

So, this chapter is a testimonial to Mom and a life well lived, with appreciation, love, and sadness. The chapter is also a reminder to readers with relatives and friends suffering from PD to ask for testimonies and even share them in the patient's darkest hours. What Sharon's family members and friends did and how they helped may also inspire readers to give as they can in any way they are moved to. Sharon profoundly appreciated what her family and friends did for her; I'm sure current sufferers will, too.

Family

Ellen: Mom's Sister

My reaction when I first heard that my sister Sharon had PD was this: What!! That can't be right. No one else in the entire family ever had it. I said, "What the hell are they talking about?"

Then, I needed to learn as much as possible about PD and its treatments. Yes, I looked at all the articles and textbooks I could find.

And she was worried. But at the time, we didn't know much about it. Unfortunately, we saw a movie on TV where the main character got PD. He ended up in a wheelchair, suffered, and then died. After that show, Sharon was afraid that would happen to her.

She told us her first neurologist gave her PD medicine that was given to patients who had already had PD for ten years.

I replied with as much confidence as I could that everyone was different. We took her to the doctors and did her shopping. We took her to eat and tried to make life easier and more typical.

Debbie: Ellen's Partner

Having a father and nephew who had PD, I knew we were in a fight to keep Sharon healthy. I supported Ellen, too, because I knew the news was hard on her.

While doing my chemo, I would shop for Sharon and take her to neurologist appointments—anything she needed. I tried to encourage her to exercise on her bike and eat healthy.

We did a lot for her. I took her to many kinds of appointments and took her for French toast at IHOP. I helped her with water deliveries and opened the bottles for her. I bought healthy food for her, put gas in her car, and checked the tire pressure.

Even in the last few months, we got her chicken noodle soup and chocolate cake from the deli. We visited with the dogs and brought our newborn daughter over for Sharon to see her.

My first reaction was to give Sharon a hug when I saw her. I prayed for her. She hugged me back, and I gave her all my love. I told her I was praying, and I gave her company. I always tried to give her joy and faith to keep up her strength. She told me that we were friends. She is a virtuous woman. Sharon was always thankful.

I loved Sharon like my sister; she was one of my best friends. I'm so sorry for your loss.

Dr. Paul Ackerman: Mom's Former Husband

I diagnosed it. It was devastating, but I didn't let her know that. I wanted to give her hope and knew that it could be years before she would deteriorate. I wanted to take her to all the best doctors. I tried to get her to the Mayo Clinic and Mass General at Harvard but was unsuccessful. But she was very grateful.

Elizabeth: Grether's Sister

I never knew what Parkinson's disease was until I heard the news about Sharon. I remember feeling sad and unsure of what the future might look like for her. My first thought was, "How can we fix this? Is there any cure?" Whenever I saw Sharon, I would smile and hug her. I didn't want her to notice any sadness. I thought she needed to see us as positive and hopeful.

No matter how unwell or uncomfortable Sharon felt, she always asked me how I was doing. This showed how caring and selfless she was.

She truly made me feel loved. As time progressed, I remember feeling anxious about the outcome. I thought about ways she could feel more comfortable. I knew she felt some peace having the family spend time with her and seeing the kids.

She always loved seeing the grandkids. I am thankful for Sharon and all that she has poured into her family.

Susan: Sharon's Cousin

My cousin Sharon lived in Florida, and I lived in New York, so we didn't see each other as much as we did when she lived in Brooklyn. When I came to Florida to visit her, she seemed fine. She was always slim. I don't remember her ever telling me she had Parkinson's until several years later. I was shocked and sorry to hear the news. The only person I knew who had Parkinson's was Michael J. Fox, and he seemed well for the most part, so I wasn't too concerned.

After moving to Florida and visiting with Sharon more often, I saw a decline in her health. But I still wasn't too worried. We spoke on the phone often, and she told me about some of her issues but with clarity. She seemed as though she was handling it well. When my husband developed Parkinson's, we discussed similarities, and I was still not that worried because Michael J. Fox was still functioning. So, I was sure Sharon had years to go before it got worse.

But it did. I remember going to her home with chicken soup and watching her, as her decline was very apparent. My heart was breaking. The next time I came, I brought her chocolate ice and fed her, putting a false smile on my face. She couldn't feed herself anymore.

The last time I saw her was to say goodbye. She was in a coma, but I knew she heard me, and I reminded her of many things we shared in life. With a heavy heart, I told her it was okay to leave.

I think of Sharon often and miss her terribly.

Adam: Sharon's Nephew

When I heard it, I was shocked but not alarmed, and I didn't know it was a fatal disease. I spent time with her when we would get the families together, and I talked to her on the phone and visits.

I went with her to several doctors' visits and spoke to the doctors. She was really looking for help, and although she did not get excellent care from them, everyone tried.

I thought about George. He's my cousin, and I tried to be there for him as much as possible.

I had known Sharon my whole life up until that point and spent an immeasurable number of moments with her. She had a great laugh and was someone anyone could talk to. I felt like she really listened and gave the best advice she could. She also threw me a graduation party after college because my family couldn't afford it, and I always appreciated that.

Friends
Judy: Sharon's Best Friend Since Childhood

When I first heard about your Mom's diagnosis, I knew that we had to do anything and everything possible to help her find the proper treatment. The mother of one of my coworkers was also battling Parkinson's and was seeing a doctor down Mom's way. He was very well known in the Parkinson's community. Mom did have a few visits with him, and then she saw his assistant. I don't remember why she stopped going to that office. I continued researching other doctors and treatments for her and found another prominent doctor; I believe he was in Gainesville, Florida. I know that she went to see him one time and then became quite ill from the dosage of the medication that was prescribed.

I drove down to Boca quite often to spend time with Sharon. We would go for lunch, go shopping, and then sit and talk for hours on end, reminiscing about our lives. After all, we had been friends since she was six months old, and I was a year old. Throughout our sixty-eight years of friendship, we spent thousands of hours talking, laughing, crying, reminiscing, and being there for each other.

When she passed away on January 1, 2020, my heart was broken. I love her and miss her every day of my life. May she rest in everlasting peace.

Lori: Sharon's Best Friend From New York

Your mother and I were very close, more like sisters than friends. We spoke on the phone daily and shared our innermost thoughts and secrets.

When I found out that she had been diagnosed with Parkinson's disease, I was devastated. As a nurse, I knew that this progressive neurological disorder would be the challenge of her life.

We shared the frustrations and hardships of her many doctors' visits and her using different medications and treatments, ultimately all to no avail. My heart broke for her suffering over and over again. She deserved better. She deserved more.

The last time I saw her was via FaceTime. You, George, held her tablet up to her. She was bedridden and no longer able to speak. I told her I loved her and always will. I said a final goodbye and cried and cried.

Her untimely death was tragic. She was robbed of her life by a vicious disease, and we were robbed of her. She was such a good soul.

May her memory be a blessing.

Janet: Sharon's Close Friend from New York

My friend Sharon was a one-of-a-kind lady. We lived a block away from each other in Brooklyn, New York. We spent many hours of our lives together. We bowled together and had lunch every week. We laughed, told stories about our single and married lives, and enjoyed our close relationship and friendship of almost ten years. We even went to the dentist together.

As time passed, Sharon and your family moved to Florida. I stayed in Brooklyn. We continued to talk on the phone. I saw her a few times in Florida. She told me she was feeling sick and that she was going to doctors to get some answers about her illness. Her calls to me got less and less.

I kept calling, but there was no answer. Then, one day, you, George, called me, telling me Mom was very sick with Parkinson's. My heart dropped. How could this have happened? My dearest friend was so ill, and I could not stop the progression of this deadly disease. I was only relieved she had a fantastic son who would care for this remarkable woman. Rest in Peace in God's Kingdom.

Stella: Sharon's Close Friend from Florida

She had been searching for so long for a diagnosis. Of course, I told her I was sorry to hear about her illness.

I wanted to scream from anger because she suffered so long. All I could do was keep in touch from my home in Virginia as often as I could to let her know I loved her. I came to see her as much as I could. She also called, and we tried to laugh as often as we could about life.

Sharon was a true friend and always told me the truth when we talked, no matter what.

I miss her laugh and knowing to call me before I called her. She was my sister.

Esta: Sharon's Good Friend in Boca Raton, Florida

I continued to be your Mom's friend. I think she told me about her illness before your wedding, and I took her for comfy shoes.

I visited her at a house that wasn't her main one. It had no paintings or wall décor, but there was an aide, and your Mom cried a lot.

This whole situation was a nightmare!

Grether: Sharon's Daughter-in-Law

When I heard about Sharon's PD, my first thought was that I knew nothing about Parkinson's disease. I did know that Sharon felt increasingly sick and was more and more vocal about her discomfort. I remember her not being able to stay out as long at restaurants and having to rest more. When eating out, increasingly she had less use of her hands, and her grip strength and coordination were affected.

However, her spirits were not. She was still optimistic and always available to celebrate with friends and have good times. She wanted to do more of that, like celebrating her sister's birthday, celebrating her own birthdays with close friends and family, and celebrating her grandchildren and watching them grow. She longed for that and often expressed anticipation for more wonderful times.

When I learned about Sharon's diagnosis, it was not openly discussed. I barely understood what it meant, and I heard from my father-in-law and husband that she was sick. I became more informed with time, and then I went with George and Sharon to the doctors' appointments. She always knew she had our unconditional support through her illness. She always said she didn't want to burden anyone, and we would say, Hush, you're not a burden.

I think I was in denial at first when I realized that she was sick. To me, she never seemed ill, and she always had the energy to come over, play with the kids, and go out to eat. I also didn't want anything to change in our perfect world, so it was very difficult to accept that things would change and progressively get worse.

All I could do for her every moment was support her and George by going to doctors' appointments, looking after the kids, and listening. George was more hands-on and proactive than I in trying to find answers and support for Sharon. I helped him as best as I could. For example, after her first hospital stay, when she fought a urinary tract infection and mental breakdown from dementia, George decided to arrange for physical therapy for her. He wanted her to be stronger and gain strength back. I helped him schedule the appointments for her caretaking and therapies. Sometimes, she was not up for treatment, and other times, she was. But the option was always there.

Throughout Sharon's illness journey, from finding out that she needed aides around the clock to her moving closer to us to her becoming more ill and her decline, I was in a mental state of unknowns. Sharon herself would ask everyone, why me? When will I get better? What will help me get better? It is a powerless feeling not to be able to answer any of those questions honestly. I would always say to her, with as much confidence as I could, you will get better; hang in there.

But really, I was just as lost as everyone who came and went from her house every day. The caretakers and nurses knew all too well what I knew deep down but didn't admit, and that was that Sharon's health was continually declining and her mental state was delicate. Then she stopped eating and was losing weight. I would know what these signs meant if I saw an older adult in that condition today.

Sharon never stopped fighting. She never gave up hope that she would get better, and until the end, that's all she wanted—to feel better. Sharon always responded to how she felt that day and in that moment. Her dementia kept worsening, causing her to act out unexpectedly. Her last caretaker was the sweetest person, and she never really knew the real Sharon. She only knew Sharon when she was confused, angry, and scared and not the joyful, sweet, caring person that Sharon was.

We continued to visit her with the kids, and she opened a playroom in her house. We brought over half of the kids' toys and filled the room, and the kids would play there. Sharon would come over and sit on the couch and play with them. In the living room, she would put on cartoons for them, blow bubbles outside with them, and watch them play in the backyard.

When the children came over, she always got out of bed to watch and enjoy them. I would sit with her and fill her in on what was happening with them at school and otherwise in their lives.

Sharon was loved every second of her journey by the people she loved and supported her all her life. She was celebrated and cared for, and she is never forgotten because she is sorely missed. Her presence was always cheerful and warm. She was a fantastic listener and always made you feel included. She was a second mother to me, and I miss her dearly.

* * * * * *

These remembrances and tributes attest to Sharon's caring and wonderful personality and the depths she inspired of love and friendship. Not only what Sharon did for my immediate family but also how she contributed to the lives of her other family and friends made me realize the unfairness of her illness. My grief was intense at the time and continues to this day. Although the doctors were well-intentioned, the woeful lack of information, uncertain treatments, and conflicting medical opinions strengthened my resolve to do everything I could to combat Parkinson's and help find a cure.

Chapter 10: The Aftermath

Four months later.
May 1, 2020

I walk by Mom's house every day. It is so depressing, sad, and empty. . . . I lost my best friend, and a piece of me was lost with her.

Due to the coronavirus, we cannot sell Mom's house. I have to continue going back there to check on things, and I get sick and dizzy seeing the empty halls and rooms.

To think that only a few months ago, Mom was here, and although she wasn't doing well because of Parkinson's and dementia, she was still here. I still had her by my side.

But now. . . . I think about what is worse—not having her here or having her here but tortured by the disease. Of course, the best scenario would have been a cure to erase 2019 and 2020 forever.

After Mom passed, my journey may have ended as her caregiver, but my grief had just begun. The funeral was something I never dreamed would happen at that time of year. Even though she was sick and not improving, we still clung to the doctors' dictum: "You do not die from Parkinson's." And we felt she was so young. Maybe we were denying or naïve, but despite her decline, Mom's passing was a complete shock.

She was always very healthy, had had no other major life-threatening illnesses, and exercised consistently. Why, why,

why? Was it the many medications, side effects, and caregivers' lack of consistency? Did they administer the proper medications at the right doses and times?

Neither Grether nor I had ever experienced the loss of a close relative. We almost didn't know how to react and feel in an alien world. I'll never forget how alone I felt, always scrambling, and hopefully trying to find the next expert or treatment and, at the same time, always trying to ensure that Mom was as comfortable as she could be.

No one except possibly nurses, I'm sure, takes a class to be a caregiver, and I was thrown right in. The caregiving didn't end with her death; I was left with so much that it felt like the weight of the world was on my shoulders. Her affairs included her personal belongings, clothes, photos, car, home, and a lifetime of memories. It was heart-wrenching.

Clearing Out

Probably every surviving child or partner who has to deal with this scenario feels similarly. What do I do with all of this? How do I make decisions on what to keep, what to give to others, and what to discard? It's overwhelming.

But I had to plunge in. So, I went over to her house and, little by little, spent afternoons or evenings sorting through her things. I almost tiptoed from room to room, holding my breath often. Otherwise, I would have burst out in tears.

Gradually, decisions surfaced. I saved some of her items for memories and donated a lot to family, friends, and organizations for others in need. In a way, I felt comforted: Mom was still helping others even after she passed. I kept the striking blue dress she wore at my wedding, and I could still smell her perfume on it. That made it even more challenging to continue to push forward.

Even throwing out several garbage bags full of her Parkinson's medicines brought back horrible memories of Mom at the worst time ever. Determinedly, I kept trying to remember the good times before Parkinson's struck.

I never realized how many memories we had, and it hit me hard. Whether tears of joy or inconsolable loss, I was sad and lost. Above all, as irrational as it sounds, and even though I had felt this before, I was furious at Parkinson's disease. And I continued to feel like a failure because we tried everything, we could but nothing worked. However, through the dark, my mother was a fighter. And because of her spirit, she was with us as long as possible.

When I became my mother's caregiver, I looked at all the areas that I needed to support her through. From taking away her car keys because she could be a danger to herself to becoming her power of attorney to ensuring her affairs were taken care of, I found each step heartbreaking. I think no one expects to have to do those things in their early sixties, but I am grateful she and we did.

But she handled her life in such an orderly manner, so accurately, and with such meticulous planning, that the final details were a little less of a burden for me. It is incredible that even then, she thought of others and did not want us to go through her dying with even more anguish.

Wills

Mom had her will drawn up about ten years before she passed. She enumerated everything with specific instructions, including her funeral, but certainly not with Parkinson's in mind. She tried to make things as easy as possible for her family.

My background as an attorney served me well, although Mom's affairs were the last thing I wanted to use it for. According to the American Bar Association, a will provides for the distribution of specific property you own at the time of your death. Generally, you may dispose of your property in any manner you choose. This right, however, may be subject to forced heirship laws in most states that prevent you from disinheriting a spouse and, in some cases, children. My mother did have some valuables and a home, and she specified the distribution of everything—jewelry, photos, clothing, furniture, and mementos she had saved. Specific jewelry items, like necklaces, watches, and other pieces, meant a lot to Mom. She ensured they stayed in the family through her granddaughter Brooke, daughter-in-law Grether, and sister Ellen.

After she passed, it was the second time we had to pack Mom's things. Earlier, we had moved her closer to us to have her with us. While packing then, she talked about how certain things were sentimental, like how she stored her wedding dress, which she bequeathed to Brooke. This last time, though, the final time, we needed and wanted to ensure it was all distributed according to her wishes.

Probably every survivor wants their loved ones to decide on the distribution of personal items for themselves. This should be done as early as possible because late-onset dementia can set in, as it did with Mom. And if it does, it poses many challenges. In some states, the loved one may not have the mental capacity to form a legal and valid binding will, and distribution can become a battleground among relatives.

Power of Attorney

I gained the positive planning trait from my mother. I have already drawn up my own will and power of attorney for my family. According to the American Bar Association, a power of attorney gives one or more people the power to act as agents on behalf of a loved one. Power of attorney is accepted in all states, but the rules and requirements differ from state to state. The power may be limited to a particular activity, such as closing the sale of the home, or apply generally in its application.

As Mom became more ill; we decided that I would become her power of attorney, although we both thought it would never be needed. I certainly never thought I would have to face such a decision. We were wrong.

One of the most challenging days was sitting in a bank with Mom and transferring her financial assets to Grether and me. From finances to everyday living, from that time forward, I had to play a massive role in helping my mother and making sure she was cared for. Her trait of planning and thinking of others over herself says a lot about her frequent declaration that she never wanted to be a burden.

She probably didn't even want me to take over as a caregiver. Of course, it was unknown territory for me and a tremendous responsibility, but as her son, I felt it was an honor. I am the man I am because of my mother's sacrifices to give me the best. It was time to help her in her time of such great need. To this day, I still do not know if Mom realized how bad Parkinson's could be and that she would not be able to handle her affairs.

If your loved one cannot make decisions under the law due to a life-ending illness, then someone needs to step in. If no one does, outside and unrelated people may have to take over, which can get messy. For example, impersonal state regulators may make decisions not in the best interest of the loved one or family. Many painful arguments and struggles can result. I'm sure you have heard of families, and even seen movies, of families going to battle against the state and each other. These can wrenchingly alienate the remaining family members, often for decades. It is all stressful and unnecessary and can be avoided by selection and appointment of the right individual to act as a power of attorney.

We did not find ourselves in this combative state because my mother planned so well, and specified everything, and she and I agreed that I would serve on her behalf. She trusted me, and despite my being an attorney, my judgment was not affected. I upheld her wishes as best I could under the law. If I had not, the state could have stepped in.

Parkinson's has no plan, time, or way to prevent or fix it. It can strike at the age of sixty, forty, or any point in an individual's life without a warning. It is crippling, debilitating, and horrific to the victim and anyone it touches in the victim's circle. It can destroy loved ones trying to figure out how to fix what has been broken but who encounter only failure at every step.

Parkinson's is an illness where the *person breathes but cannot truly live*. Towards Stage 5, they cannot participate in life; they cannot smile, cannot laugh, cannot move, cannot walk, cannot speak, cannot eat on their own, cannot enjoy their kids and grandkids, cannot enjoy their favorite music, movies, or life at all. They have nothing to look forward to and no possible future.

But they are forced to continue by lying in bed all day and night, lifeless, futureless, and without hope because there is no cure and no turning the disease around.

I did not understand anything regarding PD when I discovered my mother had the illness. And the question keeps nagging me: What else could I have done to improve her quality of life and elongate her time with us?

I realize individual caregivers have different ways of coping with Parkinson's disease when a loved one is diagnosed. I chose one way. And the entire experience set me on a journey that will never stop or end until a cure is found. Because of what my mother and our family suffered, I do not want any individual to suffer like she did or another family to have to endure what we did. And I don't want any caregiver to feel as I did—lost, afraid, and alone with so many unanswered questions.

Fighting Back

People in this world are of different types. I am a fighter. When I set my mind on things, I get them done. Despite a cure for PD being too late for us, I did not want to disappear and give up. In my despair, I discovered a new, unwavering strength. After my job duties, during Mom's illness I devoted myself to researching books and articles, searching throughout the Internet, consulting with medical professionals, and advocating. Yes, these efforts helped me deal with my grief, but they also helped me learn about the complexities of Parkinson's, the latest research, and the stories of countless others wrestling with the disease.

My efforts brought into my life a whole new world of inspiring individuals who were also fighting and never giving up until we find a cure.

And so, I became an advocate. I share my sad story to tell others and advocate for awareness because we can reach a cure with enough attention and noise. I started by sharing my mother's story, my family's journey, and the impact Parkinson's had on our lives. I've gone out into the world, speaking at local events, writing articles for newspapers, contacting experts, interviewing many touched by PD, and inspiring others with my passion and determination.

I've organized fundraisers with other dedicated individuals to support research for a cure. I've met scientists and researchers who are tirelessly working to unravel the mysteries of Parkinson's. I continue to pour my heart into these efforts, resolved to honor my mother's memory by making a difference for others battling the same disease.

Through my advocacy and the power of storytelling, I believe I have helped change the narrative around Parkinson's disease, bringing awareness not only to the physical challenges faced by those with the illness but also to the emotional toll it takes on everyone involved.

Although my mother is no longer physically present; I carry her spirit with me every step of the way. I know that one day Parkinson's will be conquered. I believe that Sharon's legacy will live on, not only through the shared memories but also through the positive changes she inspired.

Even in the face of adversity, my ongoing journey serves as a reminder that love, dedication, and the power of storytelling can spark a flame of hope that illuminates the path toward a better future.

A New Beginning

Grether and I started the website www.togetherforsharon.com as a family to keep alive my mother's memory and share messages of Parkinson's awareness and hope for a cure. If one person shares the website with another, the word will spread. If the growth so far is any indication, I am certain that more people will join the cause.

We mounted the website almost immediately after Mom passed on January 1, 2020, and in only a few months we had over 30,000 supporters. Mom would be here if we had a cure, and I will never give up on PD sufferers and their families. Her memory will live on through them.

As I shared my story, started the blog, and recounted experiences, thoughts, and feelings on social media, and people responded and continue to respond. They have been incredibly supportive and have often kept me going. We developed many warm relationships, and I now count so many like family.

There is truly no end to my journey until there is a cure discovered for Parkinson's disease. There also will never be an end to my mother's journey because, despite her passing on January 1, 2020, she will live on through me, my family, and her grandchildren.

So, a new chapter began. It was a new journey, but I was alone in this one. Reflecting again this past year, I wrote a letter in memory of Mom on December 18, 2023, two weeks before the anniversary of her passing.

* * * * * *

This time of the year is the most difficult for me, approaching the anniversary of my mother's passing from Parkinson's disease. She had no other health issues. I miss our talks, her laughter, her care, and much more than words can describe. She will always be my hero. She sacrificed throughout her life to help me become who I am today.

As her caregiver, I saw a brave young (sixties) woman go from independent, strong, and self-sufficient to utterly dependent on others. She lost all abilities, mental and physical, and even accurate memories. Now I try to forget all these and cherish only the positives. But that final year, especially the last weeks, is embedded in my mind and plagues me. What Parkinson's does to both the diagnosed and the caretaker is unimaginable.

Fifteen years ago, we had little research. I had no knowledge or awareness of what Parkinson's was. I am still not sure if my mother did not want me to know of her escalating symptoms because she didn't want to be a burden (which she never would have been) or if she, too, was unaware. We never had a chance to use some of the tools available today to slow the progression, like fitness, movement, and diet.

So, on January 1, 2024, I will visit her grave, talk with her, laugh, and remember, even though it is different. Then I think of all the caregivers today and those diagnosed with PD—so much inspiration and hope are gradually becoming reality in 2023 and beyond. And I continue to fight. I fight for everyone else because it is too late for us. It is never too late for others, and I promise never to rest until a cure is found.

This letter is not only about my mother but also about my journey. It is about us all. Together. A thank you to all those who support me and share your journeys for awareness. I call you friends and, yes, family. Your support and openness are the only things that keep my heart pumping and push me to fight for everyone worldwide. Together, our voices can shine across the world. We must be together in this!

Please hug one another, spend time together, and enjoy the time together. Have no regrets . . . .

* * * * * *

Today, I give many talks, address summits, and conduct podcasts in which I recall memories of Mom (more in these activities in the next chapter). During the talks, whether recorded or live, I can get through the challenging parts to benefit the cause of Parkinson's awareness. However, despite my tough exterior and being in the law enforcement field, I often leave the event and walk into the next room, hug my wife, and cry . . . . I miss my mother every day, and to relive my days as a caregiver as she fought Parkinson's disease is still heart-wrenching.

I keep thinking, Why Mom? The question echoes in my mind and down through the years. She didn't deserve what she suffered through. Then, I try to erase the horror of the final years with the many magical moments as I grew up, and I am so grateful for the times we were able to have. Here are some: When I was a child, walking through Disney World, seeing Broadway for the first time, the nights we all piled into a car and drove to Madison Square Garden in New York City to see life-changing performances of artists like Frank Sinatra and Whitney Houston. Mom always wanted me to experience life to the fullest. One of our favorite passions together was Broadway. We saw many plays, but our favorites remain *Phantom of the Opera* and *Fiddler on the Roof*. We had so many incredible times that Parkinson's will never take away from us.

I will continue to be an advocate in memory of my mother, Sharon Riff Ackerman, for awareness and hope for a cure until I cannot function. Please, please, join me at https://www.togetherforsharon.com

Help me prompt, stir up, stimulate, and bring a cure into being, and **NEVER** let her memory be forgotten!

Chapter 11: The Mission Forward

In 2023, as the website and related social media grew, I realized they were not only about my family's journey but everyone's throughout the world battling life-changing Parkinson's disease. Today, togetherforsharon.com® has grown worldwide, and I have interviewed over 500 individuals. Many were diagnosed with PD and are living with it, both celebrities and "regular" people. Others, who may also have PD, are caregivers, physicians, leading scientists, researchers, and others in many fields. Still others are advocates for organizations and institutions.

I keep discovering new fighters throughout the Parkinson's community, and they are all willing to share their experiences and thoughts in the hope of a cure. As I've repeated, it is too late for me and my family, but my mother lives and shines through others. Today, the only journey that is not told is the one that needs to be shared—because every journey matters.

Relationships

My dedication and these activities have led me to many new relationships with individuals going through Parkinson's, from those recently diagnosed to many who have had it for decades. I have learned of countless events and activities to raise awareness and more. I have been honored to attend and participate in walks and other events for numerous foundations and organizations. I have raised over $17,000 in four years through our website and several social media sites created in memory of Mom. These are on Twitter/X, LinkedIn, Facebook, Instagram, YouTube, and Tik Tok. We have had tables and distributed our memory bands (see below) at the American Parkinson's Disease Association's Optimism Walk, and the Parkinson's Foundation's Moving Day, held yearly in South Florida. And we continue to support these and other events.

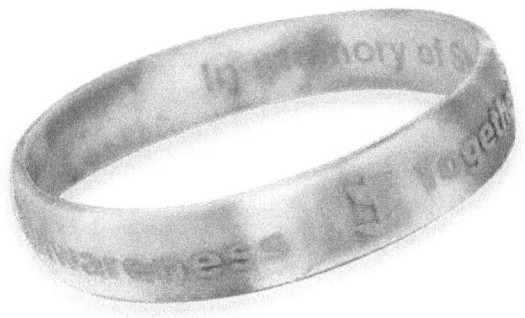

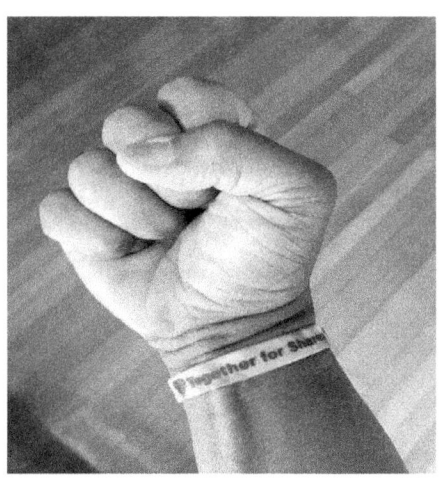

At these events, we are always touched by so many struggling with PD and their relatives and friends. They come over, hug us, and thank us for all we do, and their thanks, tears, and testimonies mean so much.

In this journey, I have had some incredible mentors, role models, and friends who have come from tragic situations. I have received invitations and spoken at meetings, conferences, and summits worldwide as an advocate for Parkinson's disease awareness. I've also been on interview shows, radio shows, videos, and television, and have had articles written about my family. All these have been in areas I never dreamed of, and all to tell Mom's and my story. I have never accepted money for any appearance or mention, and all donations go to organizations that assist with research for a cure.

Grether and I have formed relationships and partnerships with officers of foundations and organizations worldwide, giving them publicity on TogetherForSharon® without charge. When I was going through the most challenging times and searching for help, I could not locate information or programs. A great deal of information was scattered around, and no site or directory had gathered them in one place. I resolved to remedy this confusion, so I put everything I found in one area on the website, as clearly and concise as I could list it all, for others to consult and access.

Speaking

I have spoken in front of city councils and commissions and received proclamations in my mother's name for Parkinson's awareness day and month. One example: On August 22, 2023, I gave a speech to the Palm Beach County (Florida) Board of Commissioners, who then issued a Proclamation declaring August as Together for Sharon month.

I had the honor of speaking to my local U.S. representatives to assist in the history-making bill, The National Plan to End Parkinson's Disease. A special thank you to Congressman Paul Tonko and all the United States Representatives who supported and passed the bill through the House in December 2023.

Hopefully, this bill will go to the United States Senate soon because the bill and its provisions are urgent for those diagnosed with Parkinson's and caretakers, as well as researchers and scientists trying to find a cure. I have gained confirmation that my two Florida Senators are supporting the bill—and I would not have taken no for an answer if it had been otherwise. This Plan is spearheaded by the Michael J. Fox Foundation, whose members have worked rigorously to ensure the bill becomes law. It will support those diagnosed, help caregivers, and assist with groundbreaking government-funded research toward a cure. No previous legislation has ever been proposed to assist those in the Parkinson's community. To be a part of this historic law was a dream come true for me.

Publications

Sharon's and my story has been published in several magazines that feature Parkinson's awareness, research, and the experiences of patients who are coping with the disease (see Appendices). Publications began in 2020, the year of my mother's passing. The editors generously supplied room for photographs of Mom at different times in her life, of her and me, and of our bracelets. I intend to continue placing articles in magazines about Parkinson's and other debilitating illnesses, all to widen the circle of awareness and urgency for a cure. On invitation, I also recently joined AlzAuthors.com, an organization that promotes awareness of Alzheimer's, dementia, and related illnesses.

I am so grateful that many organizations like this are extending invitations to include the critical topic of Parkinson's disease advocacy. The mission of AlzAuthors.com is to continue to broaden the "community of authors who support [the site's] Mission to provide resources to light the way for those on the Alzheimer's and dementia journey."

Many organizations may not have been aware that Parkinson's is the fastest-growing neurodegenerative disease in the world. Other organizations that deal with related illnesses have not included Parkinson's in their spotlights or possibly do not have an advocate to speak out for those struggling daily with the diagnosis and the caregivers. This disease is an epidemic, and we need all those both inside and outside the Parkinson's community to band together for a cure. We are all a family in this fight. It is a universal issue that everyone should support, and there is no downside to supporting advocacy toward a cure.

Highlight

On February 2, 2024, I drove to Orlando, Florida, to meet and talk with Michael J. Fox at the MegaCon convention. This was a thrill, and I am very thankful to the organizers for this opportunity. Michael is an award-winning actor who was diagnosed with Parkinson's in 1991 when he was 29. In 2000, he founded the Michael J. Fox Foundation to raise awareness and funds and accelerate research for a cure. Remarkably, he has kept working as an actor, specifying that PD be incorporated into his roles. Michael J. Fox is a legend.

What a dream come true and honor! I explained to him that my Mom passed due to PD but that everything we all do for advocacy is driven because of his courage. I gave Michael a TogetherForSharon® band in memory of Mom (he is wearing it in the photo below) and told him that he is my hero and the entire Parkinson's community loves him.

The visit went too fast, and my heart was racing. The sadder side was that Michael was upbeat, but Parkinson's was apparent. He spoke quietly and did not try to hide the tremors. These symptoms could have been due to the timing of medications, or I may have misinterpreted something. However, his symptoms reminded me again of my mother, and I was even more saddened to see him having to fight this disease.

I felt again the overwhelming loss of my mother to Parkinson's and the terrible empathy for so many individuals I have met over the years, whom I consider friends and family and who are still struggling with this disease. And I felt a recurring sense of urgency to keep advocating even more because I am convinced that if more people were aware of PD, we would already have a cure.

When I realized that Michael had learned about togetherforsharon.com and Mom and about our efforts to support the Michael J. Fox Foundation, including Team Fox (part of Michael's foundation) and all related foundations, tears came to my eyes. They may have been tears of joy that Mom would be remembered and known by Michael, but also, I was reminded of what the disease did to her, what it does to people today whom I know and don't know, and the devastation it can still cause. All of this motivates me to get right back to advocating.

Meeting Michael was a moment engrained in my mind, heart, and soul forever. I am so thankful to you, Michael J. Fox, for never giving up on your time, dedication, and love for all those in the Parkinson's community. We send it right back to you!

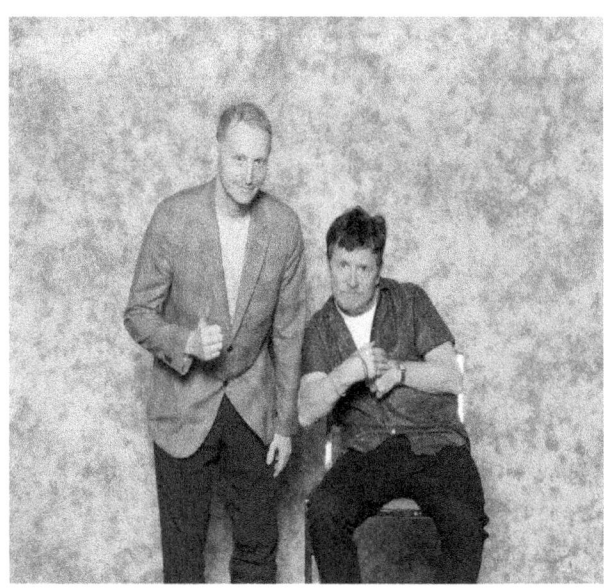

Mom's memory lives on through such meetings as this exhilarating one with Michael J. Fox, through the media, social media (Facebook, Instagram, TikTok, X, LinkedIn, YouTube—all links at https://www.togetherforsharon.com), blogs, live shows, and our story. Until a cure is found, I cannot rest, knowing so many patients, families, and caregivers are going through what Mom and I did.

As I said earlier, I feel like I am in an unusual place today. I do not have Parkinson's and am no longer a caregiver of a person living with Parkinson's. I have often felt alone, but as I became increasingly active in the many outreach activities and meet incredible people in the Parkinson's community, I no longer felt isolated. Instead, I feel blessed to have been brought into their lives, and their arms have been wide open. Words alone cannot express how much gratitude I have for everyone.

The need remains urgent for more research because Parkinson's is still difficult to understand, including its origins and individual propensities for contracting it. Some progress has been made in research, though (see below), since Mom was diagnosed, which is hopeful. If it is genetic, I may be diagnosed someday. However, as some researchers have suggested, I feel that pesticides and mold contributed to Mom's Parkinson's. She lived in a lovely home but, for many years had companies that sprayed pesticides for termites and bugs and administered chemicals for mold. Who knows what these substances do to the human body? This is only one area in which we need additional research, and we need the government to get involved to ban these poisons and dangerous chemicals from widespread use.

When I was living through my mother's PD, I realized that many in the United States had the illness, with 60 thousand people diagnosed yearly. Still, I was shocked to find out that globally, over 10 million people have been diagnosed. With these facts, the mission of togetherforsharon.com® becomes stronger: to bring awareness and provide a community for diverse people from all walks of life and throughout the world to end Parkinson's disease.

Awareness and research are growing, as is the case with the recent breakthrough of the discovery of a biomarker for PD. Parkinson's disease has gained increasing attention in the media and social media, and advocates are sharing the importance of support not only from the Parkinson's community but also now from those who do not have Parkinson's and who are not caregivers. This fight for a cure is everyone's, everywhere, local, national, and international. If we unite, our voices will be much stronger.

My emotions during caregiving were a roller coaster; I went from despair to cautious hope, thinking we had found an answer or at least some relief. Then I plummeted to an even more profound despair as my hopes were constantly dashed. More and more, I feared the worst, that Mom would be taken from me, and I faced some of the darkest days I've ever had in my forty-six years. I think of Mom daily and know she is always with me. Today, she lives on too through all the people we meet and support and who support and inspire me.

A Sustaining, Bittersweet Memory

One of my most memorable moments with Mom, and one that helps keep me going, was at my wedding. She was so proud of me, loved Grether, and knew we were right for each other. When I was growing up, Mom listened to Barry Manilow all the time and loved him. I chose his song "I Am Your Child" for our mother-son wedding dance. Despite Parkinson's, at that time Mom could still dance with me to that song. Time stood still, and nothing else mattered. Here are the lyrics:

I Am Your Child
Barry Manilow

I am your child
Wherever you go you take me too
Whatever I know, I learned from you
Whatever I do, you taught me to do
I am your child

And I am your chance
Whatever will come, will come from me
Tomorrow is won by winning me
Whatever I am, you taught me to be
I am your hope, I am your chance
I am your child

Whatever I am, you taught me to be
I am your hope, I am your chance
I am your child.

*George and Mother Sharon at George's Wedding to Grether,
December 18, 2011*

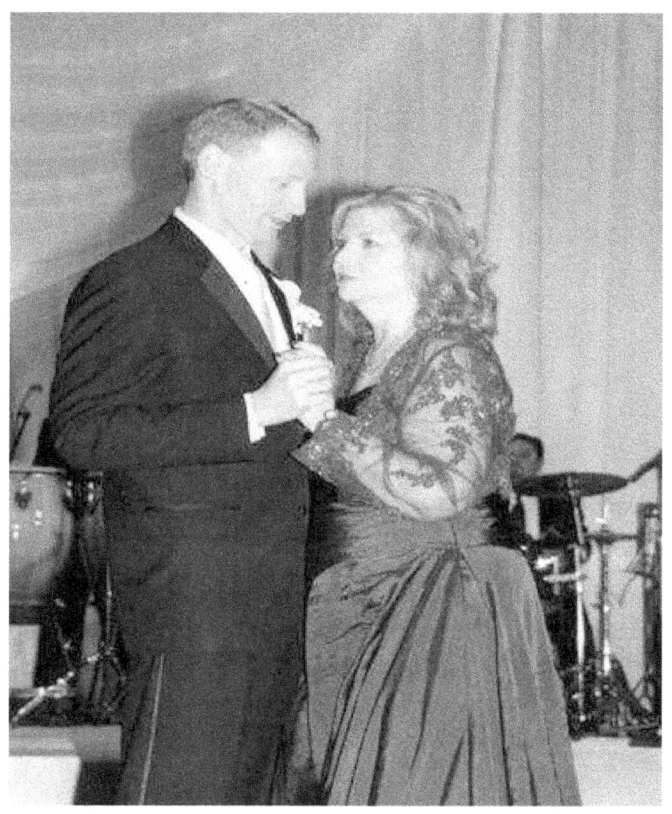

Continuing Onward

I can hardly believe Mom is no longer nearby, and I cannot go to her for her thoughts and reassurances. I often think about others going through what Mom and I did. And I cannot sleep many nights. There is still so much I want to do through advocacy for Parkinson's awareness.

And I am constantly learning. Despite the degrees, research, and experience, I learn so much from each person I meet, each challenge I hear of, and each journey people share.

But I cannot rest until I know there is a cure for others. If Mom were here, she would joke and say, "George, go spend time with your family instead." But, Mom, if you can hear me now, I love you and will never give up on ensuring you are never forgotten. We still have so much more work to do to save others.

My goal is for everyone to know they are NEVER alone! I end every article, blog, interview, and podcast with these words: "I swear that until there is a cure, I will never rest."

Ongoing Support Groups: Something Is Missing

People like me who lost a loved one due to PD are often forgotten. Yes, there are support groups for grief, for widows and widowers, for parents who have lost children, and now a few for PD victims and caregivers. But none for those who have suffered the loss of a relative (or friend) from PD. Many in the PD community welcomed me, but I have discovered organizations that just don't seem to care about PD victims once they pass or give attention to their remaining relatives and caregivers.

One organization I wanted to volunteer with; so, I started to apply on their home page; but to my surprise you must have PD or be a caregiver of a person with PD *who is alive*. I see this repeatedly. And I find it saddening. Shockingly, any organization purportedly for those with PD and their families' disregards those who lost the battle and the caregivers who still fight to ensure their memories are never forgotten. People who lost a loved one deserve a seat at the table and seem almost forgotten by many in the PD community. This needs to change.

I won't help that organization much in the future. But I already have a plan to flood social media with the message that no PD sufferer will ever be forgotten, even if they have passed. And their families and caregivers will be welcomed. Once again, we can never give up and throw in the towel. We must always make our voices heard; those we have lost should be remembered because they still matter. It was not their fault that they were not able to be here for a possible cure, and it was not their fault they were diagnosed with PD.

Despite my mother's passing, my voice can help just as much as others'. She will always have a voice through me as long as I can fight. Because someone loses the battle doesn't mean their life is no longer celebrated.

So, I ask all of you, whatever your status and connection to PD, to share and speak out. Whether past, present, or future, every life affected by PD matters to me.

What You Can Do

To join the fight, you can do many things. First, see togetherforsharon.com for a vast collection of interviews, resources, and other materials.

Then, contact your local representatives to support legislation for funding science and research to end Parkinson's disease. Keep fostering and spreading awareness through social media and word of mouth to family and friends. Volunteer at local events and fundraising walks and other activities to support those diagnosed and caregivers of people with Parkinson's. Read all you can and talk about PD whenever and wherever you can.

Rest assured, I will never stop fighting for you and countless others until a cure is found.

To those diagnosed with PD, their families, friends, and all involved I advocate for you and in memory of all those who lost their battle due to PD and their families who still want their loved one's memory to live on forever, I pledge this:

We love you; we support you, we care about you, and you are never alone!

I will continue to advocate for you.

Together our voices are so much stronger!

And I am just getting started!

Chapter 12: Grateful To So Many

It may be strange to devote an entire chapter to thanks. I do so not out of self-aggrandizement but to show and share my heartfelt appreciation for the contributions of so many people from all walks of life who have contributed to this book and my advocacy.

Advocating for a PD cure is not and cannot be a solitary effort. Many people must believe and join the undertaking—it can even be called a crusade. With increasing numbers, public opinion and laws can be swayed. Of course, researchers, scientists, and doctors work tirelessly to break through. At the same time, with advocacy awareness and belief, the collective, cultural, prevailing mindset can be swayed positively from fatalism to hope to actualization of a cure.

Thank you to everyone for your support over the years. You have all been like family and have provided so much heart and kind comments, which have never failed to uplift me and spur me on. I have gained a great deal of information and have become friends with many who have also had life-changing experiences and have provided so much to the community.

In developing and expanding togetherforsharon.com®, I have met, worked with, and become close to numerous incredible people in the Parkinson's community and organizations. I can hardly thank you all. Some influential and essential individuals who mean so much to me including: Amy

Adaniel, R. Bernard and Denise Coley, Ruth Derbin-Knowles, Coleen Greenhalgh, Larry Gifford, Esther Labib-Kiyarash, Melissa Marie Livingston, Karen Lopez, Laura Louizos, Kristina Magana, George Manahan, Desirae Mearns, Mark Milow, Dan O'Brien, Deb Pollack, Margaret Preston, Jeanne Quinn, Donna Rajkovic, Bethany Richards, Lance A. Slatton, Betsy Sloan, Cindy Surman, Karl Sterling, Matt Verguson, Stephen Williams, and A. C. Woolnough. These are not the only people; many more have become friends and family and brought a life-altering and ever-tragic loss to my darkness and grief and hope for others and light.

Interviewees

I have interviewed over 600 people, and more all the time. All have all been generous with their time and knowledge and wonderfully open about their struggles. I have a special place in my heart for them. They have had such a significant impact on me as they fight back and advocate with me.

These people include those with and without Parkinson's, those who have been suffering for a little time or a lot, people with families and without, officers of organizations and foundations, doctors, researchers, and caregivers. They are also musicians, lawyers, truck drivers, artists, doctors, businesspeople, and those in so many other fields, and they have often had to resign or take a leave due to this disease.

Researchers, Physicians, and Scientists

The knowledge I have gained from researchers, physicians, and scientists has changed my life forever. Many have written books, and some have been kind and gracious enough to speak to me about their world-changing research. These people include Bastiaan R. Bloem, M.D., Ph.D.; Ray Dorsey, M.D.; Michael S. Okun, M.D.; and many more. Thank you for your time, knowledge, and support.

Organizations and Foundations

I have made lifelong friendships and continue to share our journeys and work with people in organizations and foundations. They inspire me every day. Some include those who allowed me to interview them for awareness. They will forever hold a special place in my heart. The list is long of organizations and foundations who always have supported me: the American Parkinson's Disease Association, the Parkinson's Foundation, the Michael J. Fox Foundation: For Parkinson's Research, Team Fox, Team Fox Detroit, the Public Policy and Advocacy division of the MJFF, Drive Toward a Cure, Power Over Parkinson's, World Parkinson Congress, PD Avengers, the Brian Grant Foundation, the David Phinney Foundation, the Young Onset Parkinson's Network, PushUps4Parkinsons, Gray Strong Foundation, Punch 4 Parkinson's, Tightrope Theater, PD Movers, Dan O'Brien Parkinson's Charity, Parkinson's Resource Organization, Cure Parkinson's, Yes, And... eXercise!, Power For Parkinson's, PMD Alliance, Bike Box Project, Rock Steady Boxing, Dance for PD, Parkinson Voice Project, Spotlight YOPD, All Home Care Matters, Wendy's Parkinson Journey, Live Harder, Con De Parkinson, CCF for PSP Awareness, and countless others. I am so grateful to every individual and group.

Special recognition must go to Michael J. Fox and his foundation. His passion and advocacy have inspired me, as so many others, through his acting, appearances, books, and foundation. I feel incredibly blessed to have met him in 2024 and shared our experiences. And, as the photo above shows, he did me the honor of wearing my Together for Sharon remembrance bracelet.

Web Team

For invaluable help with the website, I heartily thank my website team at UltraWeb Marketing, who brought to life togetherforsharon.com. They take memories and make them alive. They take my interviews and refine the audio and video or take a podcast and create a movie-like environment. They have spent countless hours working to support me and help drive the mission of Parkinson's awareness and advocacy in my mother's memory. I am forever grateful to my web team; global reach would have been impossible without them.

My Local Community

I also thank my local community: the American Parkinson's Disease Association-South FL, Beyond Fitness Delray, Boca Ballet Theater, Creative Arts Therapies of the Palm Beaches, Dancing for Parkinson's (BBT4PD), the Marcus Institute of Integrative Health at Florida Atlantic University, and the Parkinson's Foundation-Florida, to name a few. Also, a special thank you to the city of Boca Raton and the Palm Beach County Commission for your time, support, and proclamation in my mother's memory.

Outside the United States/Globally

Another special thank you to all those incredible organizations, foundations, and people outside the United States. So many have opened their arms and hearts and shared their journeys. I have spoken with amazing, caring, and good-natured people in the Parkinson's communities in Africa, Alaska, Australia (Parkinson's Australia), Canada (Parkinson's Canada), France, Iceland, India, Ireland, Italy, Spain, France, United Kingdom (Parkinson's UK), Parkinson's Europe, and many more.

The Decision to Write This Book

I wrote my journal entries during the final year of Mom's life. I often felt alone and thought writing would help me through the very difficult times. And it did. At first, I decided not to share the entries as I wrote, but eventually, I realized it was time. I wanted others to know they are not alone in their feelings, stress, and anguish, victims, caregivers, families, and friends. To all caregivers, I send my love, support, and recognition that you are courageous warriors along with those diagnosed. For those diagnosed, I hear you, I see you, and I will never stop fighting for you.

For This Book, My Editor

When I finally decided to publish this book, I called on an excellent editor, Dr. Noelle Sterne. Thank you, Dr. Sterne, for the endless emails, talks, and editing to produce and publish this book. We have not simply released a book; we are changing the world for the better. I have been awed and grateful for your tireless efforts to help me share my journey with my mother, and you have understood my purpose. In the book, as you saw, I have endeavored to enlighten, encourage, and comfort others in the throes of Parkinson's toward a cure. The only journeys that break my heart are the ones I am unaware of. That needs to change, and my consistent and unrelenting efforts and this book will help inspire more research and conversations worldwide. Again, Dr. S., thank you.

Friends

To all my mother's friends, Carol, Diana, Esta, Geri, Janet, Judy, Lori, Louis, and Stella, thank you for your care and remembering all the good times with my mother. She often told me how much she loved her friends, and you were like family.

To my friends, Adam, David, Cory, Darrell, Eric, Jay, Jeremy, Keith, Matt, Michael, Mike, Ocean, Ron, and many more, so many thanks. Most of you were there before Parkinson's disease struck our family, and you have all been there throughout all the days I was caring for Mom until today. You were and are my strength, and I am grateful for your friendship.

To my mentor in life, Ken, and his wife, Pam. You have both been by my side for decades. Your care, love, support, and reliability have improved my life. I can always count on you for anything at any time. And more, of inestimable value, your advice throughout my life has always been on point and positive.

Finally, To My Family

To all of you, I am forever grateful. The long hours of silence, solitary editing, late nights, and weekends, and missing you because of my grief and need to share Mom's story were overwhelming at times but absolute necessities for me. And you understood.

Grandma Pauline, you taught me many life lessons I still use today. Your memory will never be forgotten and thank you for your constant love and consistent care during my life. You are missed.

Thank you to my father, Paul, and brother, Andrew. We all had a wonderful life together with Mom before her Parkinson's disease. No one knows her like we all do. The happiest times were the best I've ever had, and the most challenging times were the roughest. We will never forget her, and together we will continue to keep her flame going, her light glowing, and her memories in our hearts forever. You were both pillars of strength to me.

Thank you also to Ellen (Mom's sister), Debbie (Ellen's partner), Adam (Mom's nephew), Stacey (Adam's wife), and the children. Mom truly loved the times we all shared. Her decision to move us to South Florida to be with you all was a deciding moment, and I am eternally grateful. We had such frequent and incredible times together when she lived on Helsinki Circle in Boca Raton, and I will always cherish these memories. Thank you, too, for your love and care during the tough times.

To Joaquina (my mother-in-law), Elizabeth (my sister-in-law), and Austin (Elizabeth's husband), you are some of the closest individuals on this planet to me. I would not have been able to get through most days without you all by my side. I cherish each of you, and you are a part of who I am today. You were always there for Mom, took care of her, and loved her. I remember Mom always getting so excited to spend time with you, Joaquina, and Elizabeth. She always loved being with you during the years we all spent together. Thank you all for your reflections on Mom in Chapter 9.

To my children, the love Grandma showed you all at birth was a dream come true. Mom always wanted a daughter of her own, so when she found out that Brooke, our daughter, was coming, her face lit up with joy and a smile I had never seen before. That memory will stay with me forever. She loved you all, Brooke, Joshua, and Eli, and was so excited every time she spoke to or saw you, her grandchildren. Her favorite day was

Sunday, when she brought toys, books, and bubbles for you, and we all spent time playing together.

When we were all together, even in Mom's darkest times, she still smiled. She could concentrate on you three; it felt like the world and its misery had stopped. Mom always wanted to keep fighting and conquer the disease so she could be there for your milestones— school graduations, many accomplishments, and weddings. That did not happen, but she will always be with us in memory, and no disease will ever take her memory from us.

And to my wife, Grether—writing this brings tears of joy to my eyes. You have been my light in the darkness. I will never forget the day I introduced you to Mom, which I recounted in this book. I was so happy to see both of you smiling, laughing, and forming an unbelievable and unbreakable bond. It was filled with love, care, and support.

You have been there during the most difficult times, always by my side and always trying to figure out ways to help Mom, to make her more comfortable, and to combat PD so that she could be with us for many more years. You are my partner in life and my hero, and I am grateful every single moment for you, the person you are, and the support you have provided and continue to provide me.

You also wholeheartedly joined my fight against PD, never questioning it and always standing beside me with your roles in advocacy, podcasts, and events. You have always understood that I still feel a piece of me was gone when Mom passed, and you never questioned my feelings and always supported me. This book, my journey, and this story would not be complete without you by my side. I love you, thank you, and I am eternally grateful to you.

A Four-Year Remembrance and Letter of Heartfelt Thanks

Every year on January 1, we remember the day Mom was taken from us due to PD. January 1, 2024, was a hard day, a day that drives me never to want anyone diagnosed to have to go through what Mom did. It was a day I never wanted any caregiver to experience like I did. It was a day I am grateful for scientists, researchers, advocates, and all of you who tirelessly fight alongside me to someday end Parkinson's forever.

PD took my best friend in life, my role model, the person who raised me to become who I am and who stood by me through everything. Some may move on and concentrate on other things in life. I will NEVER stop fighting for a cure for Parkinson's, despite the fact a cure will not bring my mother back. I will not sit by and let it take others.

I have discovered millions of people living with Parkinson's throughout the world to fight for, and so I have met and talked with all the inspiring people I now consider family. The illness has bonded us from different paths, and we all share the same goal: to end PD forever. This disease has taken Mom, and for that, I will never forgive, but I am thankful for all of you.

You have all been my support through terrible times. You have been my voice when I felt alone. You have stood by my side on nights I couldn't sleep, thinking back to what else I may have been able to do for my mother but didn't. You comment, you send love, you send support. I wish I could share it all and END PD now.

None of us asked for this, but the light in the tunnel was that through Parkinson's we never expected to bond so closely as one and fight back. So that is what my life mission is now. You light a fire in me. You drive me. You are my hope.

Thank you, thank you, everyone, thank you all.

And Finally . . . . To my Mother, Sharon Riff Ackerman

Thank you, Mom.

Although you are no longer by my side, you will never be forgotten. Your memory will live on forever through inspiring others. Your love, intelligence, beauty, and care meant the world to me, and I would not be the man I am today without your sacrifices.

You cared for me, raised me, loved me, and did everything and more that a son could ever hope for from my childhood to the day you left.

Your life journey was not always easy, and I am grateful I had the opportunity to stand by your side as you were to me throughout my life. You were always there during both the good times and challenging times. I am honored to be your son. You taught me many life lessons that I will always carry with me.

I am happy we shared moments that meant everything to me, like my wedding, family holidays, and watching your grandchildren be born; I will never forget your smiles, holding each of them for the first time. Parkinson's disease will not take those memories away from me. In the end, Parkinson's disease does not define a person. Parkinson's may have taken years from us, but it will never dim my memories of you or defeat the passion I now have for advocacy.

The incredible memories you shared with your grandchildren will always be cherished. Memories of us on my first trip to Disney World, watching late-night television shows, visits to Broadway shows, having dinner at many wonderful restaurants, and talking about life. I miss those the most. So many memories, photos, and videos remain, and our family misses you every day.

Your love is my impetus for future generations. Your impact on me is now reaching the world and should set an example of a near-perfect mother-son relationship. You are my best friend and always will be, and although I lose sleep many nights, I wonder what would have happened if I knew you were no longer suffering. My selfishness wants you back here today, but I know it is unfair to have asked.

If I could go back in time, my only regret would be that I did not tell you enough how much you mean to me. My praise here and letters don't seem adequate. We think about those things once the person is no longer present.

Mom, I will advocate in your memory for a cure for Parkinson's disease so no one else ever goes through what you had to endure.

Parkinson's disease does not rest, so neither will I until a cure is found.

I love you, Mom, always . . . .

Your Son, George

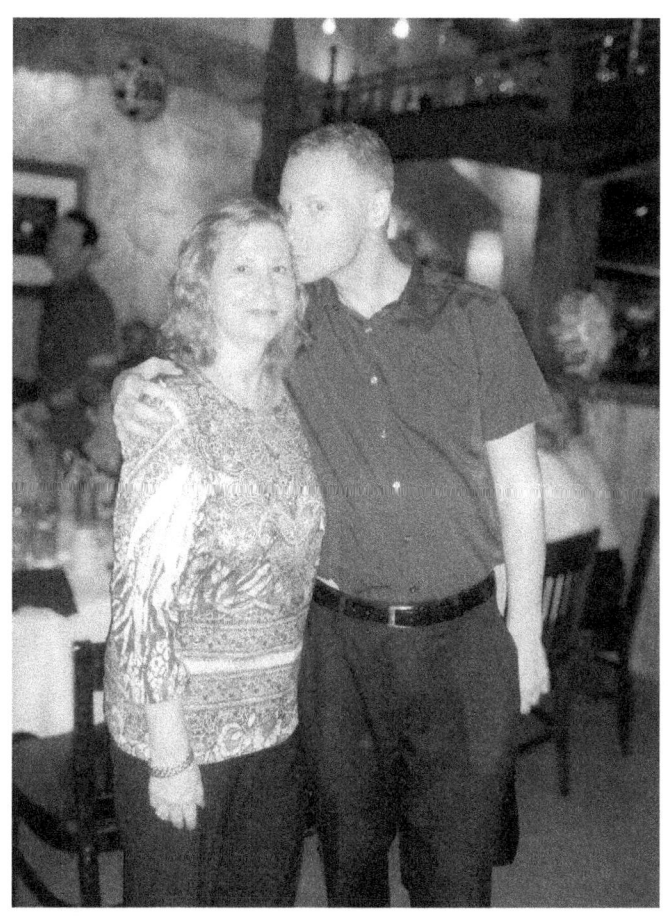

Appendices

Many books have been published on Parkinson's disease and from many perspectives. These appendices, per chapter in this book, supply selected information pertinent to each topic and especially those involving my mother. The references are not meant to be exhaustive or scholarly but contain information that helped me and may help you. More information is available in libraries with kind librarians and the Internet with similar keywords.

Chapter 1: First Signs
https://www.mayoclinic.org/diseases-conditions/parkinsons-disease/symptoms-causes/syc-20376055

https://www.parkinson.org/understanding-parkinsons

https://www.parkinson.org/understanding-parkinsons/what-is-parkinsons/stages

Chapter 2: Symptoms, Associated Illnesses, and Treatments

Parkinson, J. (1817). *An Essay on the Shaking Palsy*. Originally published as a monograph by Sherwood, Neely, and Jones (London, 1817). Reprinted 2002 *Journal of Neuropsychiatry*. https://neuro.psychiatryonline.org/doi/full/10.1176/jnp.14.2.223

Ahlskog, J. E. (2015). *The New Parkinson Disease Treatment Book*. Oxford University Press.

Temple Health. (2023). *Newly Diagnosed With Parkinson's Disease? Here's What You Need to Know.*
https://www.templehealth.org/about/blog/understanding-stages-of-parkinsons-disease
https://parkinsonslife.eu/james-parkinson-the-man-behind-the-shaking-palsy/
https://www.parkinson.org/understanding-parkinsons/what-is-parkinsons/stages
https://www.beiconicwithpd.com/
https://www.parkinson.org/

Chapter 3: My Primary Caregiving
Smith, J. (2017). *Understanding the Male Caregiver,* Home Instead Senior Care.
chromeextension://efaidnbmnnnibpcajpcglclefindmkaj/https://arch.wildapricot.org/resources/Documents/2017_National_Lifespan_Respite_Conference/Breakout_Session_PPTs/jULIE%20sMITH%20Understanding%20the%20Male%20Caregiver.pdf

Chapter 4: Steadfast Family Support: Partner
For Parkinson's Moving Day, https://www.youtube.com/watch?v=9cXsLLiuwdg&t=1s
Parkinson's Foundation: https://www.parkinson.org/
https://www.apdaparkinson.org/community/northwest/resources-support/carepartner-support-programs-resources/
PD Support Groups: https://www.parkinson.org/resources-support/carepartners/advanced/after-caregiving
https://pushups4parkinsons.org/

Chapter 5: Steadfast Family Support: Children
https://www.parkinson.org/blog/awareness/children
https://www.michaeljfox.org/news/new-guide-talking-children-and-teens-about-parkinsons

Chapter 6: Trying to Find Good Aides and Caretakers
https://www.caregiver.org/resource/parkinsons-disease-caregiving/

Search Internet with "PD in-home caregivers, PD caregiver companies/agencies, PD aides companies/agencies." Check them out with reviews.

Get personal referrals.

Chapter 7: Finally Great Caregiving
https://www.agingcare.com/Articles/best-qualities-home-health-aide-175359.htm

https://www.24hrcares.com/resource-center/caregiver-characteristics-what-makes-a-caregiver-stand-out

Chapter 8: Last Week
https://www.crossroadshospice.com/hospice-palliative-care-blog/2018/april/04/end-stage-parkinson-s-what-to-expect/

https://www.nolo.com/legal-encyclopedia/death-with-dignity-florida.html and FL law (see attached bill documented) or
https://www.flsenate.gov/Session/Bill/2023/864/BillText/Filed/PDF

The medical profession cannot tell the amount of time an individual may have until they pass on, and only specific diseases or illnesses qualify, such as terminal cancer. Parkinson's disease is not included. (Florida Bill Summary H 1231: End-of-Life Options Act)

http://www.leg.state.fl.us/Statutes/index.cfm?App_mode=Display_Statute&Search_String=&URL=0700-0799%2F0765%2FSections%2F0765.309.html

https://www.compassionandchoices.org/in-your-state/florida/bill-summary

Fl. Stat. Section 765.102 (2023).
http://www.leg.state.fl.us/statutes/index.cfm?App_mode=D

isplay_Statute&URL=0700-0799%2F0765%2FSections%2F0765.102.html

Florida Death with Dignity: https://floridadeathwithdignity.org/2023/08/02/florida-end-of-life-options-act-2023/

See "A birthday message in memory of my mother from her favorite musical artist and saxophonist Kenny G." https://www.togetherforsharon.com/celebrities

Chapter 9: Family and Friends Remember Sharon

https://everloved.com/articles/living-with-grief/ways-to-express-that-someone-is-gone-but-never-forgotten/

https://www.apdaparkinson.org/get-involved/memorial-and-tribute-gifts/

https://www.lovetoknow.com/life/grief-loss/25-creative-ways-remembering-loved-ones-at-christmas

Chapter 10: Aftermath

American Bar Association. (2024). Introduction to wills. https://www.americanbar.org/groups/real_property_trust_estate/resources/estate_planning/an_introduction_to_wills

American Bar Association, (2024). Power of attorney. https://www.americanbar.org/groups/real_property_trust_estate/resources/estate_planning/power_of_attorney/

Chapter 11: The Mission Forward

www.togetherforsharon.com

Social media:

LinkedIn https://www.linkedin.com/in/george-a-00871a82/

TikTok https://www.tiktok.com/@togetherforsharon1

Facebook https://www.facebook.com/togetherforsharon112020

Twitter/X   https://twitter.com/togetherforsha1

Instagram   https://www.instagram.com/togetherforsharon/
and threads

YouTube
https://www.youtube.com/channel/UCIeBLOelhaLQNvgeNMzu-5g
https://www.togetherforsharon.com/interview-index/

One of my appearances:
https://www.youtube.com/watch?app=desktop&v=BWvQTDsfpts
One of my speeches:
http://www.togetherforsharon.com/letter-to-congress-to-end-parkinsons/
To donate to and support the many organizations:
https://www.togetherforsharon.com/donations-fundraising/
https://www.michaeljfox.org/news/national-plan-end-parkinsons-act-makes-progress-congress
https://www.congress.gov/bill/117th-congress/senate-bill/4851
https://www.togetherforsharon.com/magazines/
https://www.facebook.com/watch/?v=659637889435891
My speech and Proclamation, Palm Beach County Board of Commissioners

My Publications:

* Moed, J. (May 29, 2020). Sharing the Message of Parkinson's Disease Awareness. *Living Magazine*.

https://www.togetherforsharon.com/living-magazine-july-2020/

* Ackerman, G. (June 27, 2023). Together for Sharon. *Insight*.

https://www.togetherforsharon.com/insight-june-2020/

* Ackerman, G. (August 31, 2023). Parkinson's Disease Awareness. *Boca Raton (FL) Tribune.* https://www.bocaratontribune.com/bocaratonnews/2023/09/parkinsons-disease-awareness/

* Ackerman, G. (2023). Together for Sharon. *Wendy van Wijk-Lugthart's Enjoying Life with Parkinson's Magazine.* https://www.togetherforsharon.com/magazines/#wendy

* Ackerman, G. (2024). Together for Sharon. *Alzheimer's Authors.*

https://alzauthors.com/

https://www.mchaeljfox.org/

https://www.scientificamerican.com/article/parkinsons-disease-and-pesticides-whats-the-connection

https://www.michaeljfox.org/publication/michael-j-fox-foundation-announces-significant-breakthrough-search-parkinsons-biomarker

Barry Manilow. "I Am Your Child." Copyright. https://barrymanilow.com/

Chapter 12: Grateful to So Many

For interviews:
https://www.togetherforsharon.com/interview-index/

For partnerships and researchers:
https://www.togetherforsharon.com/partnerships/#researcher

For podcasts:
https://www.togetherforsharon.com/podcast-interviews/

Proclamation: Palm Beach County Board of County Commissioners, Together for Sharon Month:
https://www.instagram.com/p/C0mgMIPOdl0/

About the Author

Dr. George M. Ackerman is a college professor in criminal justice, business, and law. He received his Ph.D. from the School of Public Service Leadership, Capella University; J.D. from the Shepard Broad Law Center, Nova Southeastern University; and police certification from Miami-Dade College School of Justice. His current energy is focused on advocating for a cure for Parkinson's disease through a wide range of avenues and outreach activities.

Dr. Ackerman has participated in numerous charity events; has addressed community, governmental, and international groups; has interviewed people living with Parkinson's, researchers, and advocates; has given interviews; has written about his experiences; and has participated in and conducted seminars, with plans for continued and additional activities. He also leads support groups on caregiving and loss.

Dr.Ackerman founded https://www.togetherforsharon.com/ in memory of his mother, Sharon Riff Ackerman, to increase Parkinson's awareness and research toward a cure. His dedicated interest in and passion for this work continue undiminished.

Dr. Ackerman's other interests include running charity 5Ks, basketball, and family time with his wife and three wonderful children.

In Memory of my Mother Sharon

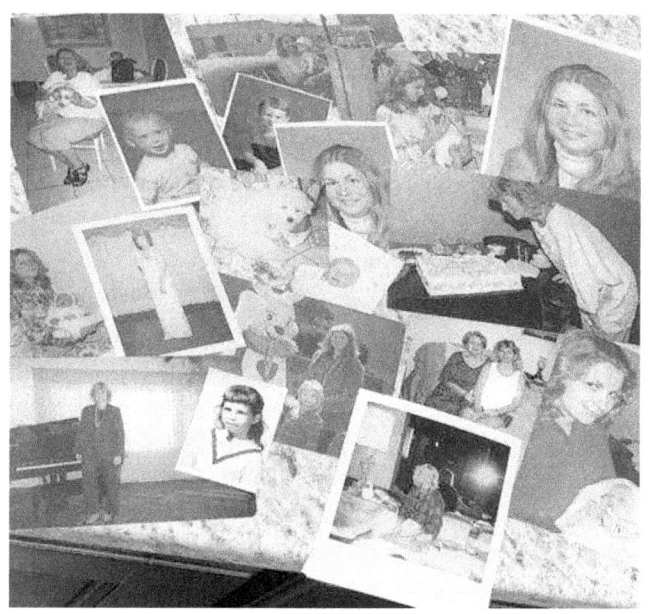

"One person can make a difference.

One person can bring positive change."

Let's keep fighting until we end PD and find a Cure!
I will be advocating right by your side.
You can count on that!

Sharon's son, George

www.ingramcontent.com/pod-product-compliance
Lightning Source LLC
Chambersburg PA
CBHW050907160426
43194CB00011B/2319